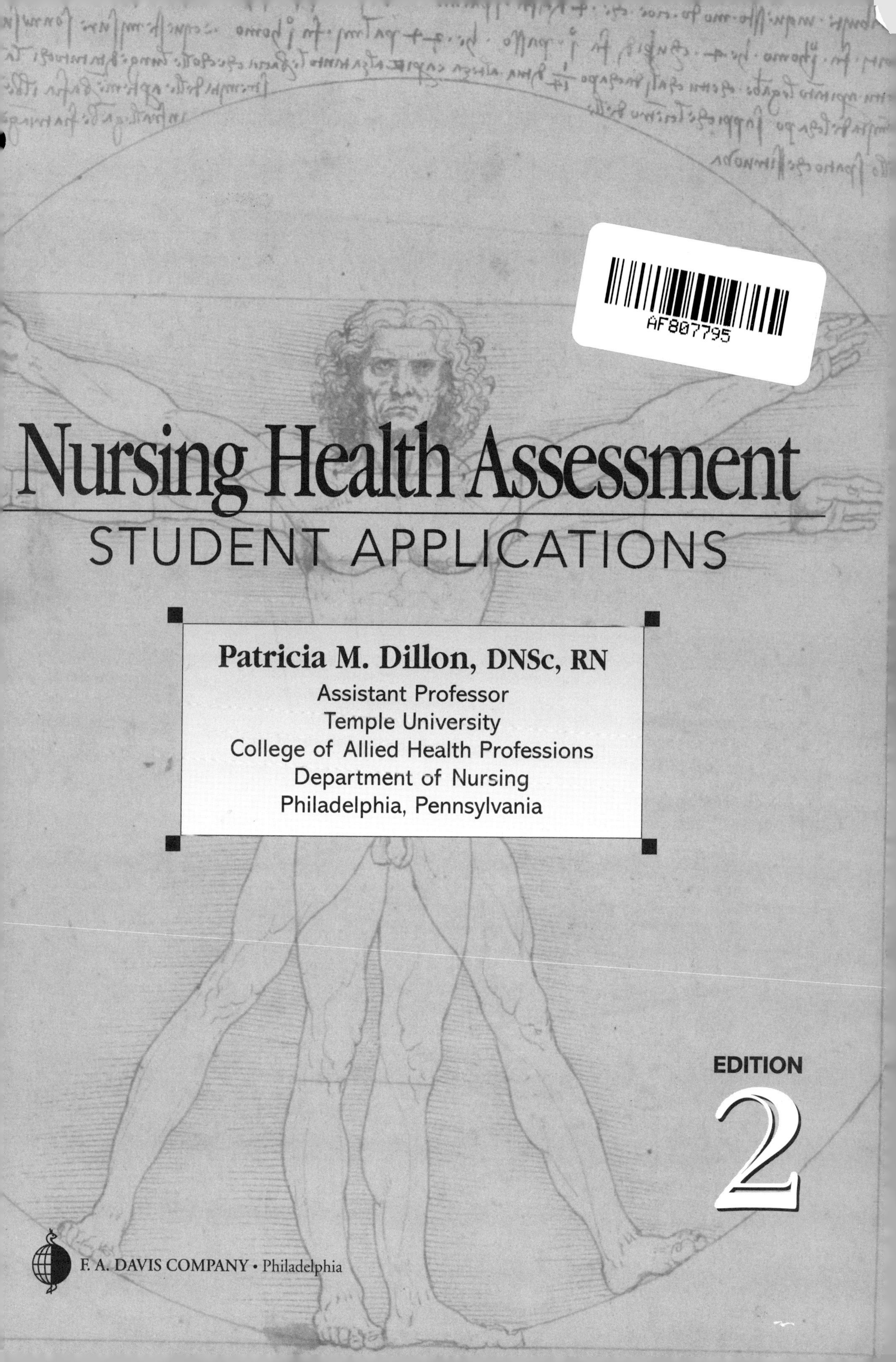

Nursing Health Assessment

STUDENT APPLICATIONS

Patricia M. Dillon, DNSc, RN
Assistant Professor
Temple University
College of Allied Health Professions
Department of Nursing
Philadelphia, Pennsylvania

EDITION 2

F. A. DAVIS COMPANY • Philadelphia

F.A. Davis Company
1915 Arch Street
Philadelphia, PA 19103
www.fadavis.com

Printed in the United States of America

Last digit indicates print number: 10 9 8 7 6 5 4 3 2 1

Publisher: Lisa B. Deitch
Developmental Editor: William F. Welsh
Production Editor: Ilysa H. Richman
Design and Illustration Manager: Carolyn O'Brien
Illustration Coordinator: Mike Carcel
Managing Editor: David Orzechowski

As new scientific information becomes available through basic and clinical research, recommended treatments and drug therapies undergo changes. The author(s) and publisher have done everything possible to make this book accurate, up to date, and in accord with accepted standards at the time of publication. The author(s), editors, and publisher are not responsible for errors or omissions or for consequences from application of the book, and make no warranty, expressed or implied, in regard to the contents of the book. Any practice described in this book should be applied by the reader in accordance with professional standards of care used in regard to the unique circumstances that may apply in each situation. The reader is advised always to check product information (package inserts) for changes and new information regarding dose and contraindications before administering any drug. Caution is especially urged when using new or infrequently ordered drugs.

ISBN 13: 9780-8036-1583-0
ISBN 10: 0-8036-1583-3

Contributors

Noreen Chikotas, DEd, CRNP, FNP
Assistant Professor
Department of Nursing
Bloomsburg University
Bloomsburg, Pennsylvania
Case study for Chapter 20. Assessing the Motor-Musculoskeletal System

Denise Demers, RN, MS
Assistant Professor of Nursing
St. Joseph's College
Standish, Maine
Case study for Chapter 17. Assessing the Abdomen

Pamela Jean Frable, ND, RN
Assistant Professor
Harris School of Nursing
Texas Christian University
Fort Worth, Texas
Case study for Chapter 6. Teaching the Client

Mary Jo Goolsby, MSN, EdD, ANP-C, FAANP
Director of Research and Education
American Academy of Nurse Practitioners
Austin, Texas
Patient Care Research Specialist
University Health Care System
Augusta, Georgia
Case study for Chapter 10. Assessing the Integumentary System
Case study for Chapter 11. Assessing the Head, Face, and Neck

Diane Greslick, RNc, MSN
Assistant Professor of Nursing
St. Joseph's College
Standish, Maine
Case study for Chapter 17. Assessing the Abdomen

Annette Gunderman, RN, EdD
Associate Professor
Department of Nursing
Bloomsburg University
Bloomsburg, Pennsylvania
Case study for Chapter 20. Assessing the Motor-Musculoskeletal System

Judith Ann Kilpatrick, RN, MSN, DNSc
Assistant Professor of Nursing
Widener University
Chester, Pennsylvania
Case study for Chapter 9. Spiritual Assessment

Carol Meadows, RNP, MNSc, APN
Instructor
University of Arkansas
Eleanor Mann School of Nursing
Fayetteville, Arkansas
Case study for Chapter 18. Assessing the Female Genitourinary System
Case study for Chapter 19. Assessing the Male Genitourinary System

Louise Niemer, RN, BSN, MSN, PhD, CPNP, ARNP
Associate Professor, Nursing
Northern Kentucky University
Highland Heights, Kentucky
Case study for Chapter 8. Assessing Nutrition

Sandra G. Raymer Raff, RN, MS, FNP
Perinatal Educator
Natividad Medical Center
Salinas, California
Case study for Chapter 22. Putting It All Together

Joanne L. Thanavaro, RN, MSN, ARNP, BC
Assistant Professor of Nursing
Jewish Hospital College of Nursing and Allied Health at Washington University
St. Louis, Missouri
Private Practice: Clayton Medical Consultants, Inc.
St. Louis, Missouri
Case study for Chapter 15. Assessing Peripheral-Vascular and Lymphatic Systems

Contents

Preface

Health assessment presents special challenges to learners, with its mass of detail that requires memorization, its organization that addresses each individual system but requires you to understand the whole, and its focus on the person as well as the body. We created this collection of activities, following the organization of the book *Nursing Health Assessment: A Critical Thinking, Case Studies Approach,* 2nd edition to enhance your learning of health assessment by:

- Providing anatomy and physiology review
- Defining a context within which you can apply assessment
- Reinforcing normal findings and selected abnormal findings
- Letting you have fun!

For each systems chapter, you will find the following:

- Normal anatomical structures that allow you to review anatomy
- A matching exercise that lets you review structure and function
- A short case study that provides a context in which you can apply assessment

Notice that the case studies within the text allow you to focus on normal, whereas we designed the case studies in the workbook to allow you to differentiate normal from abnormal.

- Short-answer situational questions that facilitate your thinking and clinical decision making
- An exercise in which we ask you to identify the relationship of the system you're currently studying and all other systems (remember to look at a specific system as a part of the whole being)
- An abnormal case study that includes a health history, physical assessment, and questions to test your critical thinking skills
- Puzzles (word searches, jumbles) to reinforce assessment content.

We hope you'll find these puzzles as fun to do as they were to create.

- A lab sheet, which covers history and physical findings and corresponds to the system chapter in the text

The history portion of the lab sheet addresses pertinent symptoms of the specific system, which you apply as they relate to that system. Review each component of the health history as it applies to the specific system being assessed. The physical assessment section of the lab sheet begins with a general survey and head-to-toe scan to identify the relationship of the particular system to other systems, then presents assessment of the system, techniques, client position, helpful hints in **bold,** alerts in ***bold italic,*** the assessment, and normal findings with developmental and cultural variations in three columns. In the fourth column, which is blank, you can document your findings as you practice on other students in lab because just as you must develop your assessment skills, you must develop your documentation skills. Include negative findings in your documentation; this will help you to remember specifics of the assessment. At the end of the lab sheet, space is provided in which you can identify pertinent history and physical findings and formulate actual or potential nursing diagnoses. (Keep in mind that you can use lab sheets as a study aid, too!)

- A self-evaluation exercise in which we ask you to identify learning achieved and further learning needed

Assessment is a skill; the more you practice, the better your skills become, and it is up to you to develop the skills and identify areas where you need more practice. Because you will be responsible and accountable for your practice and the patients you care for, so too you need to be accountable and responsible for your learning, tracking your progress and identifying further learning needs.

In Chapter 22, "Putting It All Together," complete health history and physical assessment forms are provided in which you can document your findings. We've also provided a guide "at a glance" for the health history and physical examination, which helps you perform a comprehensive systematic assessment by reminding you of questions to ask and the sequence of the examination.

Use these exercises to learn and reinforce your assessment skills. Remember, assessment is the first step of the nursing process, so make it count! Practice, practice, practice!

Chapter 1

Health Assessment and the Nurse

Name ______________________ Date ____________

Course ______________________ Instructor ______________________

1. Identify the following data as subjective or objective. Remember: Subjective data are the patient's perceptions or feelings; objective data are observable and measurable.

   - Nausea ______________________
   - Cyanosis ______________________
   - Jaundice ______________________
   - Edema ______________________
   - Numbness ______________________
   - Diaphoresis ______________________
   - Pallor ______________________
   - Ptosis ______________________
   - Dizziness ______________________
   - Stridor ______________________
   - Palpitations ______________________
   - Irregular pulse ______________________
   - Shortness of breath ______________________
   - Chest pain ______________________

2. Phyllis Johnson brings her 2-year-old daughter, Lauren, to the emergency department (ED) with a fever of 103°F. Mrs. Johnson states that Lauren has had a cough and runny nose for the past 2 days and is not sleeping or eating well. Lauren is irritable, tugs at her ear, and says "my ear hurts." Lauren's old records show that she has been treated three times over the past year for otitis media. From the data given, identify the following:

   a. Primary data source. ______________________

   b. Secondary data source. ______________________

c. Subjective data. ______________________________

d. Objective data. ______________________________

3. Match the verbal responses in the first column to the appropriate communication techniques in the second column.

Verbal Response	Communication Technique
1. "Go on."	a. Sequencing
2. "Let me see if I have this right."	b. Redirecting
3. "What does it feel like?"	c. Affirmation/facilitation
4. "You say you're afraid ..."	d. Identifying themes
5. "Getting back to why you're here ..."	e. Presenting reality
6. "From everything that you've said, it seems that you're concerned about ..."	f. Clarifying
7. "The pain started, and then what happened?"	g. General opening
8. "Remember, you're in the hospital."	h. Reflection

4. If your patient made the following statements, how would you respond?

   a. "Nurse, I have chest pain."

   ____

   b. "I'm so afraid to have surgery."

   ____

   c. "Nurse, am I going to die?"

   ____

   d. "Nurse, is it cancer?"

   ____

   e. "The night nurse made me wait all night to get pain medication."

   ____

5. The following questions/statements are common communication pitfalls. Identify the communication problem, then restate the question/statement correctly.

   a. "Does the pain go down your arm?"

   ____

   ____

   b. "In my opinion, you should ..."

   ____

   ____

c. "Don't worry, everything will be okay."

____

____

d. "You're scheduled for a laparoscopic oophorectomy."

____

____

e. "Things always look brighter in the morning."

____

____

f. "Who brought you to the hospital? And what seems to be the problem?"

____

____

g. "Don't take it out on me!" (Response to patient who says, "I can't believe I had to wait so long. This hospital is terrible!")

____

____

h. "Don't worry. Now, let's talk about surgery." (Response to patient who says, "Do you think I have cancer?")

____

____

i. "With your background, I'm sure you understand this." (Response to patient who has a Ph.D. in chemistry and is scheduled for surgery.)

____

____

j. "Maybe you should talk to your doctor. Now, let's talk about your diabetes." (Response to patient who says, "I'm really having trouble performing sexually.")

____

____

k. "What's wrong with you? If you don't take your medications, you could die." (Response to patient who doesn't take prescribed postoperative medications.)

____

____

6. Rose Montefalco, age 78, comes to the ED with chest pain. Subjective and objective data include: Patient states, “My chest is killing me; it feels like I’m in a vice.” Pain severity 10/10; difficulty breathing; blood pressure (BP) 170/110 mm Hg; pulse 118 beats/min and regular; respirations 32/min; temperature 99.8°F; pulse oximetry 90 percent on room air; patient diaphoretic, pale, and clammy; cardiac monitor shows sinus tachycardia with occasional premature ventricular contractions; electrocardiogram (ECG), chest x-ray, and cardiac enzymes done; oxygen via nasal cannula at 3 L/min. Intravenous nitroglycerin started, and chest pain decreased to 8/10 within ½ hour after starting nitroglycerin; BP 160/100 mm Hg; pulse 110 beats/min; respirations 28/min; pulse oximetry 93 percent on 3 L of oxygen. Old records show history of hypertension (HTN). From the data given, identify:

   a. Primary data source. ____________________

   b. Secondary data source. ____________________

   c. Subjective data.

   ____

   ____

   d. Objective data.

   ____

   ____

7. Document the data from question 6 using the SOAPIE method.

   ____

   ____

8. Document the data from question 6 using the DAR method.

   ____

   ____

9. Document the data from question 6 using the PIE method.

   ____

   ____

10. What’s wrong with the following documentation?

   - Mrs. Kowet, age 50
   - Past health history: Normal childhood illnesses; usual immunizations
   - Review of systems: Unremarkable
   - Psychosocial profile: Social drinker, smokes occasionally

   ____

11. Prioritize the following problems as 1, life-threatening; 2, urgent; and 3, can wait:

- BP 60/40 mm Hg. ________________
- Breathing difficulty, pulse oximetry 88 percent on room air. ________________
- Hunger and thirst. ________________
- Anxiety. ________________
- Temperature 103°F. ________________

Chapter 2

The Health History

Name ______________________ Date ____________

Course ______________________ Instructor ______________________

1. What section of the health history contains the following data?

   a. Address ______________________

   b. Contact ______________________

   c. Genetically linked problems ______________________

   d. Chief complaint ______________________

   e. Health insurance ______________________

   f. Sleep and rest patterns ______________________

   g. Immunizations ______________________

   h. Exercise patterns ______________________

   i. Menarche, last menstrual period (LMP) ______________________

   j. Hospitalizations ______________________

   k. Breast self-examination (BSE), breast masses ______________________

   l. Childhood illnesses ______________________

   m. Symptom analysis ______________________

   n. Recreation/hobbies ______________________

   o. Testicular self-examination (TSE) and prostate examination ______________________

   p. Birth date ______________________

   q. Bowel habits and laxative use ______________________

   r. Marital status ______________________

   s. Nutritional patterns ______________________

   t. General health ______________________

u. Roles and relationships ______________________________

v. Glasses, last eye examination ______________________________

w. Religion ______________________________

x. Drug and alcohol use ______________________________

y. Last chest-x-ray, purified protein derivative (PPD) ______________________________

2. Match the developmental theorists in the first column to the description of their theories in the second column.

Theorist	Theory
1. Freud	a. Moral development of individual
2. Kohlberg	b. Cognitive development of individual
3. Piaget	c. Psychosocial development of individual
4. Erikson	d. Family development
5. Maslow	e. Psychosexual development of individual
6. Butler	f. Relationship between activity and aging
7. Havighurst	g. Needs as basic to self-actualization
8. Duval	h. The elderly and life review

3. You can document family history by listing or by drawing a genogram. Document your family history as a genogram.

Chapter 3

Approach to the Physical Assessment

Name ______________________________ Date ____________

Course ____________________ Instructor ____________________

1. Match the pieces of equipment in the first column to their uses in the second column.

Equipment	Use
1. Rectal thermometer	a. Best for detecting high-pitched sounds
2. Bell portion of stethoscope	b. Detects fetal heart sounds
3. Diaphragm portion of stethoscope	c. Used to test far vision
4. Doppler	d. Most accurate means to obtain body temperature
5. Snellen eye chart	e. Best for detecting low-pitched sounds
6. Small white light of ophthalmoscope	f. Used to measure body fat
7. Transilluminator	g. Used to measure angle of joint
8. Tuning fork	h. Used to test temperature sensation
9. Triceps skinfold calipers	i. Used to test deep tendon reflexes
10. Test tubes	j. Used to visualize fontanels and sinuses
11. Hammer	k. Used to assess undilated eye
12. Goniometer	l. Used to assess vibratory sensations and hearing

2. Identify the appropriate assessment technique for the following assessment findings:

a. Organomegaly. ______________________________

b. Poor skin turgor. ______________________________

c. Resonance. ______________________________

d. Skin color changes. ______________________________

e. S_1 and S_2. ______________________________

f. Skin texture. ______________________________

g. Fetal position. ____________________

h. Floating knee cap. ____________________

i. Kidney tenderness. ____________________

j. Deep tendon reflexes. ____________________

k. Bruit. ____________________

l. Thrill. ____________________

3. Identify the part of the hand that is best for detecting the following findings:

a. Vibrations. ____________________

b. Temperature. ____________________

c. Pulsations. ____________________

4. You are assessing Barbara La Bar, age 70, who weighs 110 lb, and her husband, Leo, age 72, who weighs 250 lb. They both have normal breath sounds, but Mrs. La Bar's are louder than her husband's, which are soft and seem diminished. How would you explain the difference?

____

____

5. How should you adapt your physical assessment approach for the following age groups: Infants, preschoolers, adolescents, pregnant patients, and older adults?

____

____

____

____

6. You use different positions to assess various structures. Identify the appropriate position(s) for the following exam:

a. Pelvic exam. ____________________

b. Prostate exam. ____________________

c. Abdominal exam. ____________________

d. Spinal exam. ____________________

e. Respiratory exam. ____________________

f. Cardiac exam. ____________________

g. Rectal examination. ____________________

7. Various factors can affect accurate blood pressure (BP) readings. Identify whether the BP reading would be falsely high or low for each statement.

a. Cuff too small. ____________________

b. Cuff too loose. ____________________

c. Cuff too big. ____

d. Arm elevated above heart level. ______________________________

e. Arm muscle contracted. ______________________________________

8. Usually, either arm may be used to obtain a BP reading. Name four occasions when the use of an arm may be contraindicated.

____

____

9. How would you explain the importance of scanning every system in relation to the specific system being assessed?

____

____

Chapter 4

Assessing Pain

Name ______________________ Date __________

Course ______________________ Instructor ______________________

1. Identify the following facts about pain as truth or myth:

   a. You have to have physical signs for pain to exist. ______________________

   b. Self-report is the most accurate indicator of pain. ______________________

   c. Prolonged use of pain medication leads to addiction. ______________________

   d. Older adults have decreased pain sensation. ______________________

   e. Noncancer pain can be as severe as cancer pain. ______________________

   f. Infants have decreased perception of pain. ______________________

2. The following is a list of noxious stimuli. Identify the type as mechanical, thermal, or chemical.

   a. Surgical incision ______________________

   b. Frostbite ______________________

   c. Angina ______________________

   d. Abdominal tumor ______________________

   e. Sprained ankle ______________________

   f. Sunburn ______________________

3. Pain can be referred from the site of origin. Match the disorders in the first column with its area of referred pain in the second column.

Disorder	**Area of Referred Pain**
1. Appendicitis	a. Chest
2. Choleycystitis	b. Umbilicus
3. Angina	c. Right scapula
4. Gastroesophageal reflux disease (GERD)	d. Back
5. Urinary tract infection (UTI)	e. Jaw

4. The patient's description of pain is often helpful in identifying the type of pain. Match the descriptions of pain in the first column to the types of pain in the second column.

Description of Pain	**Type of Pain**
1. Sharp	a. Deep somatic pain
2. Dull	b. Neuropathic pain
3. Cramping	c. Superficial somatic pain
4. Shocklike	d. Visceral pain

5. Melissa Jacobs, age 45, has migraine headaches. You perform a symptom analysis to assess her pain. What questions would you want to ask?

P: ____________________

Q: ____________________

R: ____________________

S: ____________________

T: ____________________

6. Select an appropriate pain scale for the following patients:

   a. An infant being circumcised. ____________________

   b. A preschooler scheduled for a tonsillectomy. ____________________

   c. A 20-year-old scheduled for wisdom teeth extraction. ____________________

   d. A confused elderly patient with a broken hip. ____________________

Chapter 5

Approach to the Mental Health Assessment

Name ____________________ Date ____________

Course ____________________ Instructor ____________________

1. Label the following characteristics as delirium, depression, or dementia:

   a. Irreversible changes in mental status. ____________________

   b. Acute onset of changes in mental status. ____________________

   c. Behavior worse in the morning. ____________________

   d. A progressive disorder. ____________________

   e. Impaired recent and remote memory. ____________________

2. Theresa McLaughlin, 70 years old, recently lost her husband. You are assessing for additional risk factors for depression. Name five other risk factors for depression in older adults.

   a. ____________________

   b. ____________________

   c. ____________________

   d. ____________________

   e. ____________________

3. Name three physical findings that would suggest that Theresa was depressed.

   a. ____________________

   b. ____________________

   c. ____________________

4. Theresa tells you she doesn't know how she can go on. If you suspect that Theresa is suicidal, what areas would you need to assess? What questions would you ask? Name five.

   a. ____________________

   b. ____________________

c. ____________________

d. ____________________

e. ____________________

5. Theresa's loss of her husband is a situational crisis. You perform a crisis assessment. What three areas need to be addressed? What questions would you ask?

a. ____________________

b. ____________________

c. ____________________

6. Sharon Thompson, age 29, is here for her 6 week postpartum check-up. She says she has been very tired and is feeling down. You screen for postpartum depression. Identify five risk factors that would put Mrs. Thompson at risk for postpartum depression.

a. ____________________

b. ____________________

c. ____________________

d. ____________________

e. ____________________

7. You are the school nurse at a middle school. There have been reports of children playing the choking game. Name at least three findings that might suggest a child has been engaging in this dangerous game.

a. ____________________

b. ____________________

c. ____________________

8. Match the disorders in the first column with the appropriate definition in the second column.

Disorder	Definition
1. Concrete thinking	a. Repetition of words
2. Circumstantiality	b. Jumps from one topic to the next
3. Word salad	c. Misinterpretation of real external stimuli
4. Tangentialitly	d. Inability to abstract
5. Clang association	e. Digresses from topic, never getting to point
6. Echolalia	f. False belief
7. Flight of ideas	g. False sensory perceptions
8. Illusion	h. Combining words with no meaning
9. Delusion	i. Excessive, irrelevant detail
10. Hallucination	j. Association of words by sound

9. You are working in the emergency department. A patient is admitted to the emergency department after being involved in an automobile accident. The patient had been drinking alcohol. The police say this is the second driving while intoxicated (DUI) for this patient. Using the CAGE Questionnaire to assess alcohol abuse, what questions would you ask this patient?

   C ______________________________

   A ______________________________

   G ______________________________

   E ______________________________

Chapter 6

Teaching the Patient

Name ______________________________ Date ____________

Course ____________________ Instructor ____________________

1. What health history data should you use to identify your patient's learning needs and to develop a teaching plan?

____

____

2. What physical assessment data can you use to identify your patient's learning needs and to develop a teaching plan?

____

____

3. Maria Hernandez, age 50, is divorced and of Puerto Rican descent. She has a 25-year-old married son and an 18 year-old daughter who will be attending community college in the fall. Mrs. Hernandez owns her own home in a low-income neighborhood in an urban area. She is employed full-time and works 4 days a week in 10-hour daytime shifts driving a truck. She has employer-paid health insurance for herself but no insurance for her daughter. Mrs. Hernandez's son often drives her to and from work so that her daughter can use the family car to get to her workplace.

Mrs. Hernandez is 5 feet tall and weighs 225 lb. She has been diagnosed with hypertension (HTN) and non–insulin-dependent diabetes mellitus (NIDDM). According to the rules of her job, she is required to take a 45-minute lunch break and a 10-minute rest break every 1.5 hours. Mrs. Hernandez reports that she feels under a lot of pressure to make her deliveries on time, so she usually skips her breaks and grabs lunch at the drive-through of a fast-food restaurant. She also says that she doesn't like taking her "water pill" because it interferes with work and sleep and that sometimes she forgets to take her diabetes medication. She is supposed to test her blood sugar each morning with a home glucometer, but she says she does this only on the days that she is not scheduled to work.

Today, Mrs. Hernandez is complaining of lower back pain and burning and irritation on urination. Her vital signs are temperature 99°F, pulse 88 beats/min, respirations 20/min, and BP 180/100 mm Hg. Her blood glucose is 160 mg/dL. Mrs. Hernandez answers your questions, makes jokes, and tells stories during the assessment. She says she thinks that she has a urinary tract infection and needs an antibiotic so she can get back on the road. She doesn't want to lose any sick days. She says that she is saving her sick days so she can help out when her new grandchild is born next month.

From the information given, identify three areas of concern that would warrant further teaching for Mrs. Hernandez.

____

4. Identify Mrs. Hernandez's strengths that could be useful when developing a teaching plan.

____

5. Cluster the supporting data for the following nursing diagnoses.

   a. Ineffective management of therapeutic regimen related to knowledge deficit of diabetes mellitus and HTN (management and signs/symptoms of complications).

   ____

   ____

   b. Knowledge deficit regarding management of diabetes mellitus and HTN.

   ____

   ____

6. When developing Mrs. Hernandez's teaching plan for managing her health problems, what key area do you need to consider for the plan to be successful?

____

Chapter 7

Assessing Wellness

Name ______________________________ Date ____________

Course ______________________ Instructor ______________________

1. Many factors affect health behavior, including the patient's supports, psychological state, and access to healthcare. Who might be a support for your patient? How might your patient's psychological state affect his or her health behaviors? What might pose a barrier to healthcare?

____

____

2. What are *your* strengths and weaknesses regarding health and wellness? Do a self-evaluation.

____

____

3. Sleep can be affected by many factors. How might the following factors affect sleep?

- Exercise ______________________________
- Nicotine use ______________________________
- Caffeine use ______________________________
- Alcohol use ______________________________
- Weight ______________________________
- Diet ______________________________
- Stress ______________________________
- Specific medical problems ______________________________

____

4. Match the patients in the first column to the appropriate sleep patterns in the second column.

Patient	Sleep Pattern
1. Infant	a. 9–10 hr/day
2. Todder/preschooler	b. 6–8 hr/day
3. School-age child	c. 20 hr/day
4. Adolescent	d. 6–8 hr/day in segments
5. Adult	e. 10–12 hr/day with nap
6. Older adult	f. 7.5 hr/day (up late, sleeps late)

5. Horace Brown, age 75, is beginning an exercise program. Calculate his maximum heart rate and the minimum and ideal heart rate for cardiopulmonary fitness (220 − age × 60%–80%).

____

6. What sources of stress are typical for the following age groups?

- Infant ______________________
- Toddler ______________________
- School-age child ______________________
- Adolescent ______________________
- Young adult ______________________
- Middle-aged adult ______________________
- Older adult ______________________

7. What types of injuries or health problems would you assess for the following age groups?

- Infant ______________________
- Preschool/school-age child ______________________
- Adolescent ______________________
- Young/middle-aged adult ______________________
- Older adult ______________________

Chapter 8

Assessing Nutrition

Name ______________________ Date __________

Course ______________ Instructor ______________

1. Match the nutrients in the first column with their descriptions in the second column.

Nutrient	Description
1. Carbohydrate	a. Building blocks
2. Proteins	b. 60% of body weight
3. Fats	c. Major source of energy
4. Water	d. Guard against heart disease by lowering cholesterol
5. High-density lipoproteins (HDLs)	e. Provide 9 cal/g
6. Low-density lipoproteins (LDLs)	f. Major role in enzyme reactions
7. Vitamins	g. Contribute to heart disease by elevating cholesterol

2. What is the difference between water-soluble and fat-soluble vitamins?

____

3. Identify the following vitamins as water-soluble or fat-soluble:

- A ______________________________
- B ______________________________
- C ______________________________
- D ______________________________
- E ______________________________
- K ______________________________

4. Dietary requirements vary depending on the patient's age. Name one dietary requirement and its rationale for each of the following groups:

   - Infant/toddler. ______________________________
   - Preschool child. ______________________________
   - School-age child. ______________________________
   - Adolescent. ______________________________
   - Pregnant woman. ______________________________
   - Older adult. ______________________________

5. Do a 24-hour recall on yourself, evaluating your diet according to the food pyramid. Note any deficits.

   ____

6. Calculate your body mass index (BMI).

   ____

Name ______________________ Date ______________

Course ______________ Instructor ______________

Abnormal Case Study: Kim Liang

Mr. Liang, age 73, immigrated to the United States from China 5 months ago to live with his 48-year-old daughter, her American husband, and their three teenage children. His daughter has been in the United States for 25 years, and she has a profitable career in international banking. Her husband is a tax attorney. Mr. Liang's daughter has brought him to her physician to be evaluated. He was treated in China for "prostate trouble," and she is concerned that his weight loss since his arrival is due to cancer.

Health History

CHIEF COMPLAINT:

"I'm worried that my father's weight loss is due to prostate cancer."

Symptom Analysis:

P—Decreased appetite. Patient eats better when daughter fixes ethnic meals.

Q—Not applicable (NA).

R—NA.

S—Weight loss of 30 lb in past 4 to 5 months (usual weight is 175 lb); mild fatigue; denies vomiting, diarrhea, abdominal pain, dysuria, nocturia, urinary hesitancy, frequency, urgency, or dribbling/incontinence.

T—Weight loss has progressed steadily since arrival in the United States.

Current Health Status:

- Progressive weight loss from usual 175 lb to current weight of 145 lb over past 4 to 5 months.
- Patient believes weight loss is caused by decreased intake because of lack of appetite for many American foods, but is also concerned about having cancer.

Past Health History:

- Health generally "very good"; lactose intolerance since infancy; occasional cold, but never any illness that kept him from working.
- Appendectomy at age 10; corneal abrasion at age 17 incurred while playing soccer; hernia repair at age 21.
- Most significant health problem since age 21 was "prostate problem" about 3 years ago. Describes dysuria, frequency/urgency with only small amounts of urine accompanied by lower abdominal pain. Was treated with antibiotics and has had no problems since.
- Immunizations up-to-date. No additional immunizations needed to enter the United States.

Family History:

- Mother died at age 52 of breast cancer.
- Father died at age 82 of a "bad heart" (denies heart attack).
- Brother, age 78, has HTN and glaucoma.
- Sister, age 69, alive and well.
- Grandparents died of "old age."

Review of Systems:

- *General health status:* Increased fatigue over past few months.
- *Integumentary:* Skin drier than usual; blames on climate and water.
- *Head, eyes, ears, nose, throat (HEENT):* Wears glasses for reading since age 50.
- *Cardiovascular:* Denies problems.
- *Gastrointestinal:* Lactose intolerance; avoids dairy foods and uses soy-based products; daily bowel movement, brown and soft, no bleeding.
- *Genitourinary:* Denies problems; voids about four times per day, yellow urine concentrated.
- *Musculoskeletal:* Because of recent fatigue is less tolerant of physical activity (grass raking, walking).
- *Neurologic:* Denies problems.

- *Lymphatic:* Occasional colds, but has not been ill or had cold since arrival in the United States; has gotten yearly flu shot since age 60.

Psychosocial Profile:

- *Self-care activities*: Capable of full self-care, although daughter does his cooking and laundry.
- *Activity/exercise patterns:* Reads, visits museums, recently joined social group for Chinese Americans, plays cards, "talks," goes to movies, enjoys helping with yard work.
- *Nutritional patterns:* Eats three meals a day. *24-hour recall*: Breakfast—8 oz. orange juice, 1 rice cake, tea. Lunch—1 cup rice with steamed broccoli, tea. Dinner—1 cup reheated rice, $^1/_4$ cup diced chicken, $^1/_2$ cup orange sherbet, tea. Family had fried chicken (he diced some breast meat for his rice), mashed potatoes, rolls, broccoli casserole, and chocolate pie for dessert. Claims this is typical intake since being in the United States. Daughter plans meals and prepares them half the time; other family members prepare remaining meals. Some ethnic foods, but household diet is predominantly "American." Lactose intolerant—develops gas/bloating; no other food intolerances/allergies.
- *Sleep/rest patterns:* Had trouble sleeping for about 2 weeks when first arrived in the United States because of time change, but no problems at present; bedroom is removed from noise and disturbance; sleeps without awakening from about 10 P.M. to 5:30 or 6:00 A.M.; feels rested.
- *Personal habits:* Smoked for about 10 years as young adult (quit for health reasons); occasionally has plum wine on special occasions; occasional beer when in China, none in the United States.
- *Occupational health patterns:* Retired chemical engineer with "good pension."
- *Environmental health patterns:* Family lives in affluent neighborhood; large, new, two-story home with five bedrooms. Patient feels very safe.
- *Roles/relationships:* Wife died 11 years ago; has three children (son and daughter in United States, another son in England); close to daughter with whom he lives; immigrated here at children's urging. Likes son-in-law, thinks grandsons are spoiled but is very fond and proud of them. Interacts about once weekly with small group of Chinese Americans (mostly men) but prefers spending time with family. Grandsons willingly take him places and spend time with him at movies, museums, and shopping.
- *Stress/coping:* Denies much stress except when grandsons argue among themselves or with parents; uses meditation and drinks tea to relax; finds yard work especially relaxing and has assumed much responsibility for this.

7. Based on his history information, should you be concerned that Mr. Liang's weight loss is related to prostate problems? What do you suspect is the cause of his weight loss?

____

8. Evaluate Mr. Liang's diet according to the food pyramid. Are there any deficits? What are they?

____

9. Aside from the possibility of prostate cancer, what else may account for Mr. Liang's increasing fatigue?

____

Physical Assessment

- *General appearance:* Asian man, alert, attentive to questions, interacts politely and appropriately.
- *Vital signs:* Temperature 98.6°F; pulse 99 beats/min; respirations 20/min; BP 102/60 mm Hg; weight 147 lb; height 5 feet, 7 inches.
- *Integumentary:* Skin warm and dry with mild flaking.
- *HEENT:*
  - *Head:* Normocephalic with fine, evenly distributed hair; scalp dry/flaky.
  - *Eyes:* Pupils equal, responsive to light; light reflexes equal; follows object through all fields; sclerae white, conjunctivae pale.
  - *Ears:* Tympanic membranes pearly gray, normal light reflex, normal mobility.
  - *Nose:* Midline, no septal deviation, membranes pale/moist.
  - *Mouth/throat:* Dentition intact and in good repair; tongue midline, gag intact; throat pink without exudate/erythema.
  - *Neck:* No lymphadenopathy.
- *Respiratory:* Unlabored, breath sounds equal bilaterally, clear to auscultation.
- *Cardiovascular:* No visible precordial activity; point of maximal impulse not visible, palpable on midclavicular line in fifth intercostal space; normal sinus rhythm with grade 2/6 systolic murmur.
- *Gastrointestinal:* Bowel sounds present and regular, although slightly diminished; no signs of distress with palpation; no palpable masses.
- *Genitourinary:* Normal male genitalia.
- *Musculoskeletal:* Minimal muscle resistance +4/5 upper and lower extremities; full passive range of motion (ROM); extremities symmetrical, no joint swelling/inflammation.
- *Neurologic:* Cranial nerves intact; deep tendon reflexes equal, +2 throughout.
- *Hematological:* Hematocrit 38, hemoglobin 13.0.

10. Because the patient's daughter is concerned about the possibility of prostate cancer, what additional assessment is warranted?

    ____

11. Aside from weight loss and fatigue, what additional findings would you expect if Mr. Liang did have prostate cancer?

    ____

12. Mr. Liang's nutritional deficits could also result in anemia. What assessment findings suggest anemia?

    ____

13. Calculate (approximately) Mr. Liang's percent of weight change and BMI. Interpret the meaning of the values obtained.

    ____

14. Cluster the supporting data for the following nursing diagnoses.

    a. Nutritional imbalance, less than body requirements.

    ____

    ____

    b. Fluid volume deficit related to decreased oral intake.

    ____

    ____

c. Fatigue related to nutritional deficits.

____

____

15. Identify any additional nursing diagnoses for Mr. Liang.

____

____

Chapter 9

Spiritual Assessment

Name ______________________ Date ____________

Course ____________________ Instructor ____________________

1. When assessing spirituality, focus on your patient's behavior, communication, relationships, and environment. Identify spirituality assessment data for each of the following four areas:
   - Behavior. ____________________
   - Communication. ____________________
   - Relationships. ____________________
   - Environment. ____________________
2. Name six healthcare areas that might be influenced by your patient's spirituality or religious beliefs.

   ____
3. How might being Jewish affect one's health practices?

   ____
4. How might being Catholic affect one's health practices?

   ____
5. How might being Islamic affect one's health practices?

   ____
6. How might being Hindu affect one's health practices?

   ____
7. How might being of the New Age faith affect one's health practices?

   ____

Name ______________________ Date ______________

Course ______________________ Instructor ______________________

Abnormal Case Study: Concetta Ramirez

Mrs. Ramirez is a 38-year-old Roman Catholic of Mexican descent. She is being seen by the community health nurse for follow-up after a hospitalization for cervical cancer. Mrs. Ramirez had symptoms related to her cancer for several months before seeking medical care. Her family consults a healer known as a curandero (male) or curandera (female) for most illnesses. The curandero views illness from a religious/spiritual and social context, rather than from the Western medical-scientific perspective.

Although she has received nutrition counseling, Mrs. Ramirez will not eat the foods the nurse tells her are important to aid in healing. Mrs. Ramirez states, "I got sick because I sinned. It is right that I suffer."

Health History

Biographical Data:

- 38-year-old, married woman, mother of four children, ages 4, 7, 15, and 17.
- Married for 20 years. Husband, Carlo, works for the city as a maintenance supervisor.
- Born in El Paso, Texas, of immigrant Mexican parents.
- Moved to Philadelphia with husband 12 years ago.
- Has health insurance through husband's employment.

Current Health Status:

- Recently had surgery for cervical cancer.
- Scheduled for follow-up radiation therapy to begin 6 weeks after surgery.
- Tired most of the time and has difficulty completing household tasks.

Past Health History:

- Gravida 5, para 4 (one stillbirth).
- Hospitalized for burns of lower legs 5 years ago after a cooking pot spilled from the stove.

Psychosocial Profile:

- *Typical day:* Arises at 6 A.M., makes breakfast for husband, packs his lunch. Gets children up for school, makes breakfast, packs lunches for them. After three older children leave, has cup of coffee, makes beds, washes dishes, and straightens house. Lately, needs to rest frequently as she works. Older children have been helping with younger ones. Patient finds it hard to keep up with Ramon, the 4-year-old.
- *Activity/exercise patterns*: Patient tries to lie down during the day but finds it difficult because of Ramon. Climbing the stairs in their three-story row home is all the exercise she can tolerate.

Spiritual Assessment

NONVERBAL

- When nurse makes home visit, patient rarely speaks unless questioned.
- Patient appears anxious, pacing the floor and wringing her hands.

VERBAL

- Patient acknowledges that her illness is God's punishment for a sin.
- Speaks of stillbirth of her middle child, who would be 12 years old now, as another punishment.

ROLES/RELATIONSHIPS

- Speaks of love for her husband and the strength she takes from him.
- Many family pictures in living room.
- Shows concern for her children's future and is proud of their accomplishments in school.

ENVIRONMENT

- Crucifix over each doorway in home.
- Small shrine of Blessed Virgin Mary in a sheltered place in tiny front yard.
- Patient fingers rosary beads during home visit.

ADDITIONAL QUESTIONS/ANSWERS

- Who are your support people? "My family gives me strength to go on. I don't know what I would do without them."
- Besides your family, do you have any other support? "After I attend Mass I feel better and able to face life. Father Angelo helps me."
- What gives your life meaning? "Being able to cook and keep a clean house for my family. Being a good parent to my children and a good wife for Carlo."
- How has that changed since you became sick? "It is harder to keep up with the cooking and cleaning. The older girls help, but I want them to do good in school. It's hard to be a good mother to them in this neighborhood. There are so many temptations."

8. What religious/spiritual concerns of Mrs. Ramirez's should you be aware of?

____

____

9. What cultural concerns should you be aware of?

____

____

10. What spiritual needs does Mrs. Ramirez have?

____

____

Chapter 10

Assessing the Integumentary System

Name ______________________ Date ____________

Course ____________________ Instructor ____________________

1. Anatomy review: Label the following structures:
   - Stratum corneum
   - Stratum lucidum
   - Stratum granulosum
   - Stratum germinativum
   - Connective tissue
   - Eccrine sweat gland
   - Artery
   - Vein
   - Adipose tissue
   - Arrector pili muscle
   - Hair follicle
   - Apocrine sweat gland
   - Dermis
   - Sebaceous gland
   - Hair shafts
   - Epidermis
   - Subcutaneous tissue
   - Stratum basale
   - Stratum spinosum

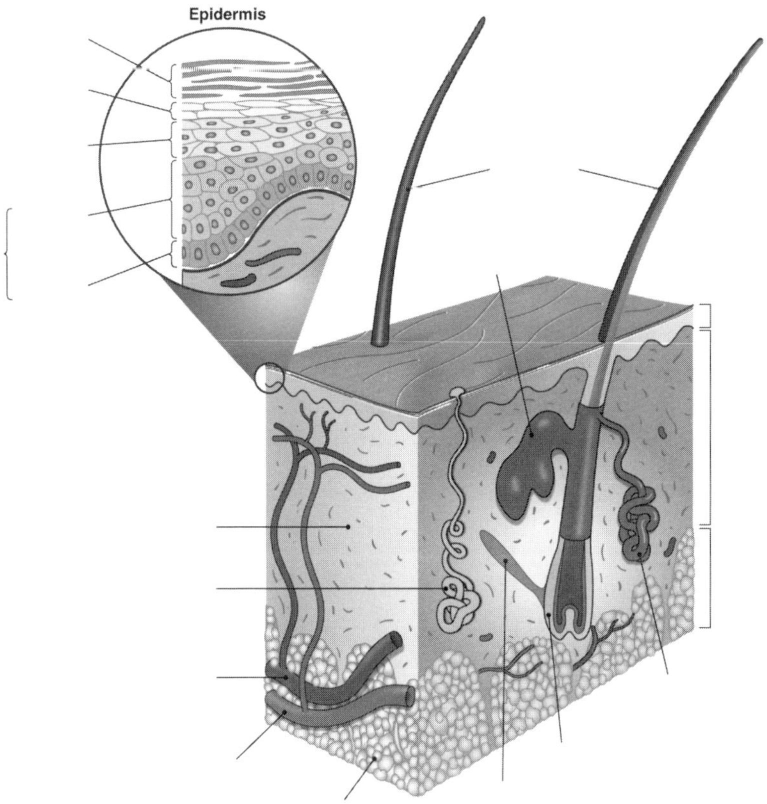

2. Match the structures in the first column to their specific functions in the second column.

Structure	Function
1. Epidermis	a. Translucent layer of dead cells found only on palms of hands and soles of feet; prevents sunburn
2. Eccrine glands	b. Produces new cells and melanin
3. Stratum corneum	c. Outer protective layer of skin
4. Apocrine gland	d. Continually produces new cells to replace worn-off cells
5. Dermis	e. Produce sebum, which lubricates and protects skin and hair
6. Melanin	f. Keratinized layer that prevents loss or entry of water
7. Ceruminous gland	g. Adds strength and elasticity to skin
8. Subcutaneous layer	h. Secretes ear wax
9. Arrector pili muscles	i. Keratinization begins at this layer
10. Lunula	j. Determines pigmentation
11. Stratum lucidum	k. Cause goose bumps
12. Stratum granulosum	l. Contains connective and adipose tissue
13. Stratum basale	m. White proximal part of nail
14. Sebaceous glands	n. Secretes sweat; helps control body temperature
15. Stratum germinativum	o. Secretes pheromones; found in axillae and genital area

3. Mr. Janewsky is admitted to the hospital with the diagnosis of acute exacerbation of chronic obstructive pulmonary disease (COPD). You are assessing him for signs of hypoxia. How would you assess and differentiate central cyanosis from peripheral cyanosis?

____

____

4. You check Mr. Janewsky's nails for clubbing. How would you describe clubbing?

____

____

5. You are working at a health fair performing skin assessment screenings for skin cancer. Mary Kane, age 75, Irish and fair-skinned, asks you to check a lesion on her arm. She is concerned that it might be skin cancer. List five questions you should ask that will help you identify Mrs. Kane's skin cancer risk factors.

____

____

6. You inspect the lesion on Mrs. Kane's arm. List at least five characteristics that you should include in a morphological description of the lesion.

____

____

7. Considering Mrs. Kane's age, what skin, hair, and nail changes would you expect to find as a normal outcome of aging?

8. Identify four common skin lesions seen with aging.

9. What four characteristics of a skin lesion indicate a malignancy and warrant referral?

10. Besides describing Mrs. Kane's skin lesion, what five additional skin characteristics should you include in her skin assessment?

11. How would you assess color change for someone with dark skin?

12. Mrs. Kane also says that she seems to be losing hair. List five history questions that might be related to her hair loss.

13. Even though your assessment focuses on the integumentary system, all systems are related. What assessment findings (subjective or objective) show the relationship between the integumentary system and other systems?

Name ______________________ Date ______________

Course ______________ Instructor ______________

Abnormal Case Study: Sheila Long

Sheila Long is admitted to the medical unit with a primary diagnosis of pneumonia. She is 86 years old and lives with her daughter because she needs help with all activities of daily living (ADL). For several months, Mrs. Long has been confined to bed. Her daughter reports that over 3 days, Mrs. Long became increasingly confused and agitated and had a temperature averaging 100.8°F. Then, during the past 24 hours, she became extremely lethargic and had little urine output. Her daughter brought her to the emergency department, and Mrs. Long was admitted and put on intravenous antibiotics.

Health History (Obtained from Daughter)

Current Health Status:

- Patient appears to be in state of gradual decline. Shows less and less interest in what is going on around her and is confused, often not recognizing relatives. Daughter rarely gets her out of bed because she is afraid patient will fall.
- Daughter has noticed reddened areas on both heels and buttocks and has been "rubbing these aggressively to ensure good circulation."

Past Health History:

- Patient's only major diagnosis is senile dementia.
- Has been hospitalized six times in the past 3 years for urinary tract infections and pneumonia.
- Before the past few years, patient was never hospitalized. Her only childbirth was uncomplicated and occurred at home.
- Has no known history of allergies.
- Has no history of specific skin disorders, including eczema, psoriasis, seborrhea, or skin cancer.
- Because the patient does not leave the home and is never directly exposed to infections, daughter wonders how the patient keeps getting sick.
- Immunizations include a pneumonia vaccine 3 years ago and an annual flu shot.
- Takes no medication.

Family History:

- Daughter unsure of what problems led to maternal grandparents' deaths, but says that they lived into their 70s and seemed in good health until very near death.
- Patient had three siblings, with only one sister (age 81) still alive. Sister has history of breast cancer but otherwise lives independently in apparent good health. One brother died of a heart attack at age 59, and the other died in a car accident as a youth.
- Daughter is an only child and has hypertension (HTN) and depression, both well controlled.
- Patient has four grown grandchildren who live out of state and are all in good health.

Psychosocial Profile:

- *Health practices:* Receives a thorough bath 3 days/wk, when a home health aide comes to assist. Daughter gives her a quick sponge bath on other days. No self-care activities.
- *Typical day:* Spent in her bedroom. Daughter awakens her at 8 A.M. to change her diaper and feed her. Patient naps on and off throughout the day. TV is often on, and her daughter often talks to her about other family members and current events, although patient rarely responds.
- *Nutritional patterns:* Eats three meals a day, taking fair portions as long as she is fed. Daughter admits she doesn't encourage her to drink because patient previously had aspiration pneumonia.

- *Activity/exercise patterns:* Daughter performs range of motion (ROM) exercises on patient's arms and legs twice a day for 10 minutes. Other than that, only activity is spontaneous movement in bed.
- *Sleep/rest patterns:* Usually sleeps through the night.
- *Personal habits:* Takes no prescribed or over-the-counter (OTC) medications unless she has an acute illness. Has no intake of caffeine or alcohol and has never smoked.
- *Environmental health patterns:* Daughter knows of no environmental exposures. Daughter's home is one-story and climate-controlled. Patient's bedroom is bright and airy, with large windows.
- *Roles/relationships:* Patient occasionally responds to her daughter or son-in-law, but has little interaction otherwise. Occasionally, a neighbor or member of her church visits, but she does not recognize them.

14. What factors from Mrs. Long's history place her at risk for integumentary problems?

____

____

Physical Assessment

- *General appearance:* Lethargic; frail appearance consistent with stated age; slender, with wrinkled, loose skin; inattentive to environment.
- *Vital signs:* Temperature 101.2°F; pulse 116 beats/min, regular; respirations 28/min with slight effort; blood pressure (BP) 112/68 mm Hg.
- *Integumentary:*
- *Skin:* Warm and dry; turgor poor, with tenting evident over forehead, upper arm, and upper chest; loose and thin, with many wrinkles; coloring extremely pale pink; no visible freckles and few moles; all moles < 0.5 cm and medium tan; 9 to 10 scattered small red papules, all < 0.5 cm (cherry angiomas). Four raised brown lesions (seborrheic keratoses) with well-circumscribed borders and rough surface texture with "stuck-on" appearance. Surrounding skin intact and consistent with general coloring. Three lesions on upper back and one on right upper anterior chest. All are 2 to 3.5 cm in diameter. Both heels have a 2-cm reddened area that remains 30 minutes after heel pressure is relieved by placing pillows beneath lower legs. Epidermis intact. Reddened area, 3 cm, over sacrum, with a 2- to 3-mm area of central denuding.
- *Hair:* Completely gray and sparse, yet evenly distributed, clean, long, and in braid; scalp easily visible, pink, without lesions; several coarse, gray hairs along chin line.
- *Nails:* Long, but edges smoothly filed; nailbeds faintly dusky blue, firm to palpation; no hemorrhages evident; no clubbing.

15. What factors from Mrs. Long's physical assessment place her at risk for integumentary problems?

____

____

16. Considering Mrs. Long's age, what assessment findings might be considered a normal part of aging?

____

____

17. Cluster the supporting data for the following nursing diagnoses:

    a. Impaired skin integrity related to effects of pressure.

    ____

    b. Fluid volume deficit related to restricted oral intake.

    ____

    c. Total incontinence related to confusion.

    ____

18. Identify any additional nursing diagnoses for Mrs. Long.

    ____

    ____

19. *Word search:* Find the following lesions in the puzzle: crust, cyst, erosion, keloid, macule, mole, papule, purpura, pustule, scar, tumor.

B	R	A	D	D	I	O	L	E	K	R	E
P	U	M	A	P	U	S	T	U	L	E	C
U	T	S	M	A	A	T	U	M	E	T	K
R	S	C	A	P	R	Y	M	O	S	E	P
U	M	A	C	U	L	E	O	S	I	K	Z
P	O	R	Y	T	P	C	R	C	O	T	S
K	L	E	S	E	R	O	S	I	O	N	M
T	E	U	T	S	U	R	C	R	U	S	T
E	R	P	U	R	P	U	R	A	P	U	T
C	U	S	C	M	M	E	L	U	P	A	P

Name ______________________________ Date ______________

Course ______________________ Instructor ______________________

Student Lab Sheet: Integumentary

Client's Initials: ______________________

Age: ______________________

Gender: ______________________

Health History

BIOGRAPHICAL DATA:

Current Health Status:
Symptom Analysis (PQRST):

- Changes in moles or other lesions
- Nonhealing sore or chronic ulceration
- Pruritus/itching
- Rashes
- Hair changes
- Nail changes

Past Health History:

- Childhood illnesses
- Hospitalizations
- Surgeries
- Serious injuries/chronic illness
- Immunizations
- Allergies (food, drugs, and environmental)
- Medications (prescribed and OTC)
- Recent travel/military service

Family History:

Review of Systems:

- General health status
- HEENT
- Respiratory
- Cardiovascular
- Gastrointestinal
- Genitourinary
- Musculoskeletal
- Neurologic
- Endocrine
- Lymphatic/hematological

Psychosocial Profile:

- Health practices and beliefs/self-care activities
- Typical day
- Nutritional patterns (24-hour recall)
- Activity/exercise patterns
- Recreation, pets, hobbies
- Sleep/rest patterns
- Personal habits (tobacco, alcohol, caffeine, drugs)
- Occupational health patterns
- Socioeconomic status
- Environmental health patterns
- Roles, relationships, self-concept
- Cultural/religious influences
- Family roles and relationships
- Sexuality patterns
- Social supports
- Stress/coping

Physical Assessment

GENERAL SURVEY:

- Vital signs
- Height
- Weight

Head-to-Toe Scan:

- HEENT
- Respiratory
- Cardiovascular
- Abdomen
- Genitourinary
- Musculoskeletal
- Neurologic

Assessment of the Integumentary System

Area/Physical Assessment Skill	Assessment	Normal Findings Developmental/Cultural Variations	Student's Findings
INSPECTION	**Compare side to side throughout exam**		
Skin	Note color, odor, integrity. Differentiate central (mouth and conjunctiva) cyanosis from peripheral (extremities) cyanosis. **Cold or hot weather can affect surface characteristics of skin and nails.** **In dark-skinned patients, look for color changes in conjunctiva or oral mucosa.** Identify any primary, secondary, or vascular lesions. Describe morphology, distribution, pattern, location. **Assess for malignant lesions** **A = Asymmetry** **B = Border irregularity** **C = Color variation** **D = Diameter > 0.5 cm**	Uniform skin color with slightly darker exposed areas. No jaundice, cyanosis, pallor, erythema, hyper-/hypopigmentation. Ethnic/racial differences account for many variations in color. Mucous membranes and conjunctiva pink. No unusual odors. Skin intact, no suspicious lesions.	
Hair and scalp	Note color, quantity, distribution of hair, condition of scalp, presence of lesions or pediculosis. **Gender, genetics, and age affect hair distribution.** **Puberty marks onset of pubic hair growth with increased hair growth on legs and axillae.**	Hair evenly distributed over scalp, no alopecia. Normal balding patterns common to men and elderly. Hair color appropriate; thins and grays with age. Fine body hair (vellus) noted over most of body. No lesions or pediculosis.	

Nails	Note color, condition, angle of attachment, presence of focal or generalized abnormalities (e.g., ridges, clubbing).	Color varies from pink to light brown in darker-skinned patients. Nails well groomed and convex. Cuticle pink and intact. Angle of attachment 160 degrees.	
PALPATION	**Maintain standard precautions.** **Wear gloves if assessing an open area.**		
Skin	Temperature **(use dorsal part of hand).** Turgor **(test unexposed area, e.g., below clavicle).** Texture, hydration **(exposed areas tend to be drier).** Palpate for tenderness and surface characteristics of any lesions. Check for pulsations and blanching of vascular lesions.	Skin warm and dry. Moisture depends on body area. Positive turgor, no tenting. Texture varies from soft/fine to coarse/thick depending on area and patient's age. Skin coarser on extensor surfaces. Older adult skin may be drier, coarser, thinner with decreased turgor and increase in lesions.	
Hair	Palpate scalp for tenderness, masses, and mobility. Note texture of hair.	Scalp mobile, nontender. Hair texture varies (fine, medium, coarse) depending on genetics and treatments (e.g., permanents).	
Nails	Texture and capillary refill.	Nails smooth and firm; no ridges; adhere well to nail bed. Brisk capillary refill < 3 seconds.	

Assessment of the Integumentary System (continued)

Pertinent Health History Findings:

Pertinent Physical Assessment Findings:

Nursing Diagnoses (Actual or Potential) With Clustered Data:

Name		Date	
Course		Instructor	

Self-Evaluation Exercise

Integumentary System	Yes	No	Need More Practice
1. Applies knowledge of integumentary system anatomy and physiology in performing an integumentary system assessment.			
2. Applies growth and development principles as applicable to the integumentary system.			
3. Considers cultural variations as indicated when performing an integumentary assessment.			
4. Gathers all equipment necessary to perform an assessment of the integumentary system.			
5. Obtains history specific to assessment of the integumentary system.			
6. Performs a physical assessment of the integumentary system, including: • General survey and head-to-toe scan. • Inspection. • Palpation.			
7. Documents integumentary assessment findings.			
8. Identifies normal/abnormal findings.			
9. Clusters pertinent subjective/objective data.			
10. Identifies actual/potential health problems and states them as nursing diagnoses with supporting data.			

Chapter 11

Assessing the Head, Face, and Neck

Name ______________________________ Date ____________

Course ____________________ Instructor ____________________

1. Anatomy review: Label the following mouth and neck structures.

   a. Upper lip
   b. Gingiva (gum)
   c. Hard palate
   d. Soft palate
   e. Glossopalatine arch
   f. Pharyngopalatine arch
   g. Palatine tonsil
   h. Uvula
   i. Posterior pharyngeal wall
   j. Papillae of tongue
   k. Lower lip

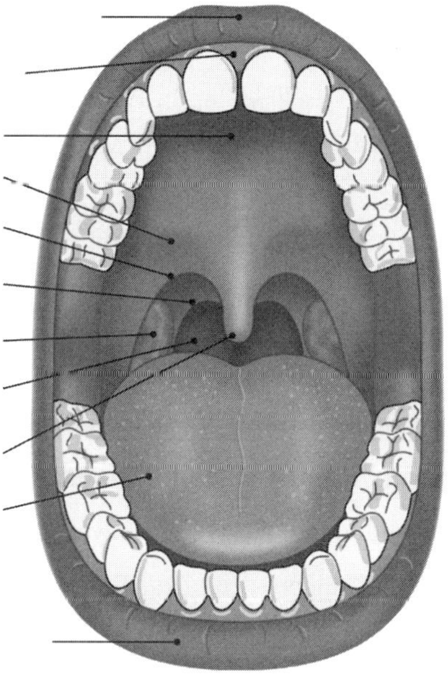

   a. Hyoid bone
   b. Thyroid cartilage
   c. Cricoid cartilage
   d. Isthmus
   e. Right thyroid lobe
   f. Left thyroid lobe
   g. Trachea

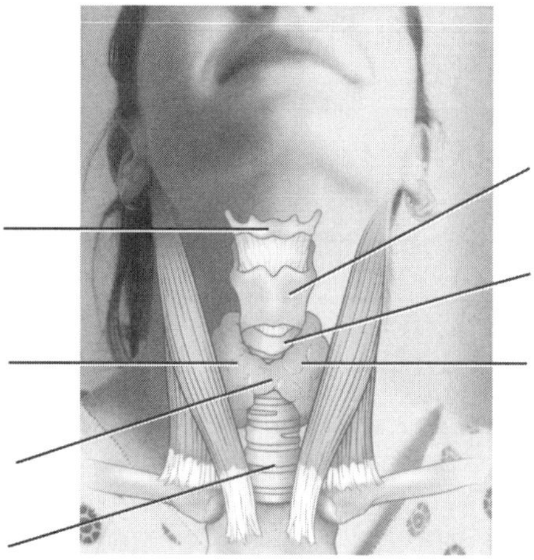

a. Occipital
b. Posterior auricular
c. Preauricular
d. Tonsilar
e. Submandibular
f. Submental
g. Superficial
h. Deep cervical
i. Posterior cervical
j. Superclavicular

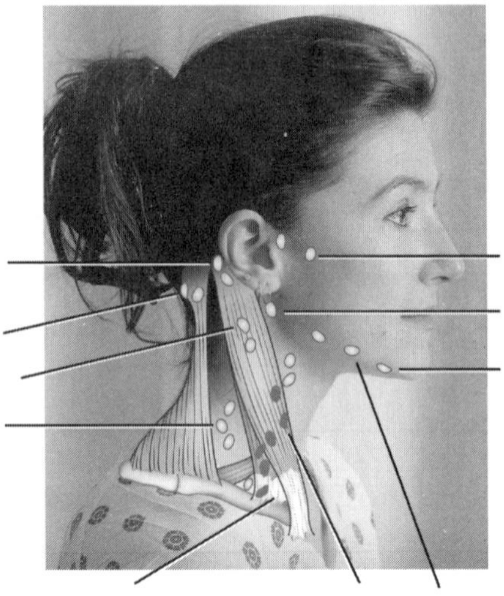

2. Match the structures in the first column to their specific functions in the second column.

Structure	Function
1. Paranasal sinuses	a. Control metabolism
2. Buccal mucosa	b. Air cavities that add resonance to voice
3. Gingiva	c. Lymphatic tissue that prevents infection
4. Cilia	d. Mucous membrane of cheeks
5. Uvula	e. Drain saliva from parotid glands
6. Turbinates	f. Small hairs that filter air
7. Tonsils	g. Anchors teeth
8. Soft palate	h. Increase nasal surface area to filter, warm, and humidify air
9. Salivary glands	i. Produce saliva
10. Thyroid gland	j. Prevents food from entering nasal passages
11. Stensen's ducts	k. Drain saliva from submandibular glands
12. Wharton's ducts	l. Prevents food and saliva from entering nasopharynx

3. Mrs. Hunter says that her 4-year-old son Jared has had a sore throat and fever for 2 days and that today he complained of an earache. When inspecting Jared's throat, what three things might you expect to find?

____

4. Considering Jared's age, how many teeth would you normally expect to find?

____

5. Name three characteristics you should note when inspecting the teeth.

____

6. What three characteristics should you note when inspecting Jared's gums?

____

7. Jared's rapid strep test is positive, and an antibiotic is prescribed. Considering his age, what type of antibiotic is contraindicated and why?

____

8. You also check Jared for any lymph node enlargement, and palpate tonsillar, superficial, and auricular nodes. What characteristics differentiate normal nodes from infected or malignant nodes?

____

____

9. The anterior and posterior triangles are important landmarks when assessing the lymph nodes. What two muscles make up these triangles?

____

10. You are assessing Sue Lynch, a 33-year-old woman with thyroid disease. When inspecting her thyroid gland, what three neck positions should you use?

____

11. Landmarking is essential in palpating the thyroid gland. Where is the isthmus of the thyroid located?

____

12. The thyroid gland is usually not palpable. What are the two exceptions?

____

13. What additional assessments should you perform when assessing the head of an infant or toddler?

____

____

14. What two facial areas are best for assessing symmetry of facial features?

____

15. Although your assessment focuses on the head, face, and neck, all systems are related. What assessment findings (subjective or objective) show the relationship between the head, face, and neck and other systems?

____

____

Name ______________________ Date ______________

Course ______________________ Instructor ______________________

Abnormal Case Study: Loretta Markus

Loretta Markus, a 65-year-old African American woman, is admitted to your nursing unit after a stroke. She lives alone, and earlier today she experienced transient paralysis of her left extremities, urinary incontinence, and difficulty with her speech. After visiting the ED, she is admitted for observation and evaluation. Mrs. Markus has recovered some use of her left arm and leg, and her speech is currently intact.

Health History

CURRENT HEALTH STATUS:

Believes that she has been in "pretty good health." Says that she has been independent, able to care for herself, and able to perform all housework and yard work since her husband of 26 years died 2 years ago.

Past Health History:

- Has had hypertension (HTN) for at least 10 years. Has been out of medication for some time and has not had her blood pressure (BP) checked recently.
- Has been hospitalized only for two uncomplicated vaginal deliveries at ages 23 and 25.
- Has allergy to penicillin, which causes a generalized rash.
- Has no history of disorders involving the head, face, or neck, including hay fever, temporomandibular joint (TMJ) disorder, sinusitis, lymphoma, or thyroid disease.
- Uncertain about her immunization history, but is sure she has had no immunizations since she was quite young.
- Does not currently take any medications, but used to take hydrochlorothiazide, 25 mg daily, and propranolol, 80 mg daily.
- Experienced menopause at approximately age 50 and takes no hormones.

Family History:

- Parents both died in their mid to late 60s. Mother died of a stroke, and father died after several heart attacks.
- Uncertain of cause of death for grandparents. Knows that paternal grandfather died at fairly young age after some type of accident. Other grandparents "died of old age" in their 70s or later.
- Has three siblings, all alive: sister (age 63) and two brothers (ages 64 and 68). All have trouble with their heart or BP. Oldest brother was a heavy smoker for many years and had cancer of larynx and now "has no voice box."
- Two daughters are in good health and take no medication that she knows of.
- Has seven grandchildren, all in good health.

Psychosocial Profile:

- *Typical day:* Gets up at 8 A.M. and usually spends day working in house or yard. Daughters live nearby, and she visits frequently with her children, grandchildren, and nieces and nephews.
- *Nutritional patterns:* Eats three fairly well-balanced meals a day: cereal or toast for breakfast, fried meat two to three times a week, vegetables twice a day, some fruit daily. Lately, appetite has increased, but she believes that she has lost about 10 lb in the past 4 to 6 weeks "without really trying."
- *Sleep/rest patterns:* Goes to bed around 10:30 P.M. and has no trouble falling asleep. Usually sleeps well, but for the past few weeks has been wakeful at night and not sleeping well.
- *Personal habits:* Used to smoke cigarettes, but quit smoking when she developed HTN. About 3 to 4 years after she quit smoking, she started chewing tobacco and uses two to three packets per week. Rarely drinks alcohol—"maybe a sip or two of wine twice a year."

- *Occupational health patterns:* Used to work in a factory where electronic equipment components were made. Quit working when plant closed 5 years ago and she was unable to find work elsewhere.
- *Socioeconomic status*: Has a small pension from husband and draws Social Security. Says she is "barely able to make ends meet." Has had no health insurance for 5 years and is happy to be 65 so that she can start using Medicare.
- *Environmental health patterns:* Owns a small, one-story, two-bedroom home. Says it has two window air conditioning units and central heating, which are adequate.
- *Stress/coping:* Believes that she deals with stress pretty well. Is active in church and has a strong faith. Admits to being a little "on edge" and irritable lately, but has not been able to identify a cause.

16. Based on the information provided by Mrs. Markus, what, if any, real or potential problems related to her head, face, and neck do you recognize?

____

____

Physical Assessment

- *General appearance:* Alert, oriented; appearance consistent with stated age; slightly overweight; no apparent distress.
- *Vital signs:* Temperature 97.2°F; pulse 102 beats/min; respirations 16/min, regular and unlabored; BP 186/108 mm Hg; weight 152 lb; height 5 feet, 4 inches.
- *HEENT:*
  - *Head:* Normocephalic; no obvious deformities or lesions.
  - *Face:* Symmetry of features; slight asymmetry of movements, with motion on left side of face diminished; no deformities.
  - *Sinuses:* Nontender to palpation or percussion; transillumination not performed.
  - *Eyes:* Conjunctivae pink and moist; extraocular muscles intact and conjugate.
  - *Ears:* Hearing grossly intact; cerumen blockage bilaterally obscures exam.
  - *Nose:* Midline placement; no nasal flaring; no discharge; mucosa pink and moist; no deformities, lesions, polyps.
  - *Mouth:* Lips midline and symmetrical at rest, light brown, consistent with generalized coloring, no lesions; left weakness of lips detected with frown and exaggerated smile; full upper/lower dentures in place, removed for exam; gingiva intact, pink/moist, no erosion or lesions; 1 cm x 2 cm white patch with slight induration palpated on right buccal mucosa adjacent to right upper molars site; otherwise, buccal mucosa pink and moist with no indurations, nodules, or lesions. No visible or palpable lesions, nodules, or indurations of tongue or mucosa at floor of mouth or over palates.
  - *Throat:* Tonsils not visible; uvula midline and rises with phonation; posterior wall smooth and without lesions or drainage.
  - *Nodes:* Two right submandibular nodes, firm-to-hard, mobile, nontender, palpable; no other palpable nodes.
  - *Thyroid:* Not visible; slightly palpable bilaterally and symmetrical; meaty consistency, no tenderness or nodules.
- *Respiratory:* Breath sounds clear bilaterally; unlabored respirations; no wheezing, crackles, or other adventitious sounds; no cough.
- *Cardiovascular:* Apical and radial pulses regular at 102 beats/min; S_1 and S_2 auscultated with no murmur, extra heart sounds; mild, 1+ edema of feet bilaterally; soft bruit bilaterally.
- *Musculoskeletal:* Full range of motion (ROM); no tenderness or deformities; strength 5/5 right, 4/5 left.
- *Neurologic:* Slight slurring of some words, sensation slightly diminished on left side of face, tongue strength +4/5 to the left; otherwise, cranial nerves grossly intact. Movements of right side coordinated, with +5/5 strength. Movements of left side are slightly clumsy, with +4/5 strength.

17. What factors in Mrs. Markus's assessment place her at risk for stroke?

___

18. What assessment findings suggest transient ischemic attack (TIA)/stroke?

___

19. What factors in Mrs. Markus's assessment place her at risk for or suggest oral cancer?

___

20. Identify teaching needs for Mrs. Markus.

___

21. Cluster the supporting data for the following nursing diagnoses:

    a. Risk for altered nutrition less than required.

    ___

    ___

    b. Decreased motor function left side of face; decreased sensation.

    ___

    ___

    c. Risk for impaired communication.

    ___

    ___

22. Identify any additional nursing diagnoses for Mrs. Markus.

___

___

23. *Word jumble:* Unscramble the following words. Then unscramble the circled letters to complete the sentence: A precancerous oral lesion is called

    1. L U (K) S L
    2. D T (O) I R H Y
    3. (L) V U A U
    4. E S I (U) S N S
    5. I D C O (I) R C
    6. O (S) (L) T N I
    7. E T N B (A) R I U T S
    8. H (P) Y L M
    9. E T (E) H T
    10. I N G (A) V G I
    11. C (K) E N
    12. E O G T I R

Name ______________________ Date ______________

Course ______________ Instructor ______________

Student Lab Sheet: Assessing the Head, Face, and Neck

Health History

BIOGRAPHICAL DATA:

Current Health Status:
Symptom Analysis (PQRST):

- Headaches
- Lesions on mouth or lips
- Swelling of head or neck areas
- Difficulty chewing or swallowing
- Fatigue
- Nasal discharge or postnasal drip
- Hoarseness or voice change

Past Health History:

- Childhood illnesses
- Hospitalizations
- Surgeries
- Serious injuries/chronic illness
- Immunizations
- Allergies (food, drugs, and environmental)
- Medications (prescribed and over-the-counter [OTC])
- Recent travel/military service

Family History:

Review of Systems:

- General health status
- Integumentary
- Eyes/ears
- Respiratory
- Cardiovascular
- Gastrointestinal
- Genitourinary
- Musculoskeletal
- Neurologic
- Endocrine
- Lymphatic/hematological

Psychosocial Profile:

- Health practices and beliefs/self-care activities
- Typical day
- Nutritional patterns (24-hour recall)
- Activity/exercise patterns
- Recreation, pets, hobbies
- Sleep/rest patterns
- Personal habits (tobacco, alcohol, caffeine, drugs)
- Occupational health patterns
- Socioeconomic status
- Environmental health patterns
- Roles, relationships, self-concept
- Cultural/religious influences
- Family roles and relationships
- Sexuality patterns
- Social supports
- Stress/coping

Physical Assessment

GENERAL SURVEY:

- Vital signs
- Height
- Weight

Head-to-Toe Scan:

- General health status
- Integumentary
- Eyes/ears
- Respiratory
- Cardiovascular
- Abdomen
- Genitourinary
- Musculoskeletal
- Neurologic

Assessment of the Head, Face, and Neck

Area/Physical Assessment Skill	Assessment	Normal Findings Developmental/Cultural Variations	Student's Findings
INSPECTION	Position: Sitting		
Head	Note size, shape, symmetry, position. Assess fontanels and measure head circumference in newborns.	Normocephalic, erect and midline; molding in newborns from vaginal delivery.	
Face	Note facial expression, symmetry of facial features, abnormal movements, lesions, and hair distribution. **Nasolabial folds and palpebral fissures are a good place to check for symmetry.**	Facial expression appropriate; hair distribution appropriate for age, sex, and ethnicity; no lesions or abnormal movements. Nasolabial folds and palpebral fissures symmetrical.	
Nose	Note position, deformities, septal deviation, discharge, flaring. **Types of discharge: clear, bloody, purulent.** ***If clear drainage noted from nose or ears, secondary to head trauma, suspect cerebrospinal fluid (CSF).*** ***Nasal flaring sign of respiratory distress in newborns.*** Use nasoscope or otoscope with nasal speculum to assess nasal mucosa for color, intactness, lesions, edema, and discharge.	Nose midline, symmetrical, no deviation, no flaring. Nasal mucosa pink and moist, no lesions, edema, or discharge. Septum intact.	
Frontal and maxillary sinuses	**Frontal sinuses are located above eyebrow; maxillary below eyes.** Note periorbital edema or "dark circles" under eyes. Transilluminate sinuses if indicated.	No periorbital edema noted. Sinuses clear; positive transillumination.	
Parotid and submandibular glands	**Parotid glands located in front of ears; submandibular glands under mandible.** Note any edema, redness.	No edema or redness noted over salivary glands.	
Lips	Note color, condition, lesions, breath odor, pursed-lip breathing.	Lips pink, moist, intact, no lesions, no unusual odor (halitosis), no pursed-lip breathing.	

Oral mucosa	Note color, conditions, lesions. ***Leukoplakia or "smoker's" lesion is a white, nontender, precancerous lesion that warrants follow-up.*** Inspect Stensen's and Wharton's ducts for inflammation. **Stensen's duct located opposite second upper molar; Wharton's duct on floor of mouth under tongue.**	Oral mucosa pink, moist, intact, no lesions. Oral mucosa may be bluish or have patchy appearance in dark-skinned individuals. Stensen's and Wharton's ducts patent; no inflammation.	
Gingivae	Note color, condition, retraction, hypertrophy, edema, bleeding, lesions.	Gingivae pink, moist, intact; no bleeding, edema, retraction, or lesions. During pregnancy, gingivae may normally hypertrophy.	
Teeth	Note number, color, condition, occlusion, missing or loose teeth. ***A loose tooth could dislodge and obstruct the airway.***	32 teeth (adult), 20 (child), white, in good repair, none missing or loose. Edges smooth, no caries. Good occlusion.	
Tongue	Note color, texture, position, mobility, involuntary movements, and lesions. Mobility of tongue. **(Cranial nerve [CN] XII)**	Tongue pink, moist, papillae intact, midline with full mobility, no lesions or involuntary movements, geographic tongue normal variation.	
Oropharynx, hard/soft palate, tonsils, uvula	Note color, condition, lesions, drainage, exudates, edema. Using penlight, have patient say "ah" and look for symmetrical rise of uvula and swallow reflex. **(CNs IX and X)**	Hard and soft palate pink and intact, tonsils pink, symmetrical, +1, no lesions or exudates, symmetrical rise of uvula, positive swallow reflex.	
Neck, thyroid and cervical lymph nodes	**Inspect neck in neutral position, hyperextended, and as patient swallows.** Note symmetry, ROM, and condition of skin. Note thyroid or lymph node enlargement. **Use anterior and posterior triangles as landmarks.**	Neck and cervical lymph nodes symmetrical, active ROM, no masses, skin intact. Larynx and trachea rise with swallowing. Older patients may have limited ROM of neck.	

(continued)

Assessment of the Head, Face, and Neck (continued)

Area/Physical Assessment Skill	Assessment	Normal Findings Developmental/Cultural Variations	Student's Findings
PALPATION	**Maintain standard precautions. Wear gloves when palpating oral structures or if lesions suspected.**		
Head	Note masses, tenderness, scalp mobility. In children < 2 years old, assess fontanels and measure head circumference. **Anterior fontanel closes by 18 to 24 months; posterior fontanel by 2 months.**	Head symmetrical, no masses, nontender, scalp freely movable. For children: Note if head circumference is above or below growth norms for established growth percentile. Fontanels should be sof and flat.	
Face	Palpate bony structures of face and jaw. Note condition and symmetry, tenderness, muscle tone, and TMJ function.	Facial bones smooth, intact, symmetrical, nontender. Good muscle tone. TMJ with full active ROM, no crepitation or tenderness noted.	
Nose	Palpate for tenderness, deformity, and patency.	No nasal tenderness or deformities. Nares patent.	
Frontal and maxillary sinuses	Palpate for tenderness.	Sinuses nontender.	
Parotid and submandibular glands	Parotid glands located in front of ears; submandibular glands under mandible. Note enlargement or tenderness.	Salivary glands not enlarged, nontender.	
Lips and tongue	Palpate for tenderness, muscle tone, and lesions.	Soft, nontender with good muscle tone. No lesions.	
Oropharynx	Test gag reflex by touching back of soft palate with tongue blade. ***Absent gag reflex poses risk for aspiration.***	Positive gag reflex (CNs IX and X).	
Thyroid gland	Use anterior or posterior approach. **Locate thyroid isthmus below cricoid cartilage.** Palpate at edge of sternocleidomastoid as patient swallows.	Nonpalpable, nontender thyroid. Small, smooth edge of thyroid may be palpable. Palpable in high-output states such as pregnancy and puberty; not normally palpable in elderly.	

	Note size, shape, consistency, tenderness, and nodules.		
Cervical lymph nodes	Note size, shape, symmetry, consistency, mobility, tenderness, and temperature of palpable nodes. **Use light palpation with your finger pads in a circular movement.** **Use direct percussion.**	Nonpalpable, nontender cervical lymph nodes. Superficial nodes or "shotty" node may be palpable, small $>$ 1 cm, mobile, soft-to-firm, nontender. May normally be palpable in children; normal node $>$ 3 cm, firm, round, well-defined, mobile, nontender, symmetrical.	
Frontal and maxillary sinuses	Percuss sinuses for tenderness.	Sinuses nontender.	
AUSCULTATION	**Use bell of stethoscope.**		
Thyroid gland	If thyroid gland enlarged, auscultate for bruits while patient holds breath.	No bruits.	

Assessment of the Head, Face, and Neck (continued)

Pertinent Health History Findings:

Pertinent Physical Assessment Findings:

Nursing Diagnoses (Actual or Potential) With Clustered Data:

Name ______________________ Date __________

Course ______________ Instructor ______________

Self-Evaluation Exercise

Head, Face, and Neck	Yes	No	Needs More Practice
1. Applies knowledge of head, face, and neck anatomy and physiology in performing head, face, and neck assessment.			
2. Applies growth and development principles as applicable to the head, face, and neck regions.			
3. Considers cultural variations as indicated when performing a head, face, and neck assessment.			
4. Gathers all equipment necessary to perform a head, face, and neck assessment.			
5. Obtains history specific to a head, face, and neck assessment.			
6. Performs a physical assessment of the head, face, and neck, including: • General survey. • Inspection. • Palpation. • Percussion. • Auscultation.			
7. Documents head, face, and neck assessment findings.			
8. Identifies normal/abnormal findings.			
9. Clusters pertinent subjective/objective data.			
10. Identifies actual/potential health problems and states them as nursing diagnoses with supporting data.			

Chapter 12

Assessing the Eye and the Ear

Name ______________________________ Date ____________

Course ____________________ Instructor ____________________

The Eye

1. Anatomy review: Label the following eye structures:
   a. Eyebrow
   b. Upper eyelid
   c. Iris
   d. Pupil
   e. Caruncle
   f. Lower eyelid
   g. Eyelash
   h. Sclera covered by bulbar conjunctiva
   i. Palpebral conjunctiva covers lids
   j. Lacrimal punctum
   k. Medial canthus
   l. Lateral canthus

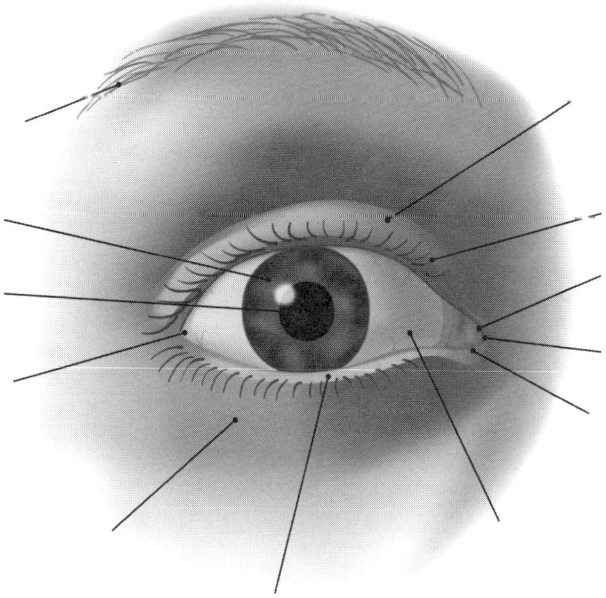

a. Cornea
b. Anterior chamber
c. Orbicularis oculi muscle
d. Iris
e. Pupil
f. Tarsal plate
g. Meibomian gland in tarsal plate
h. Orbital fat
i. Lens
j. Sclera
k. Posterior chamber
l. Ciliary body
m. Frontal bone

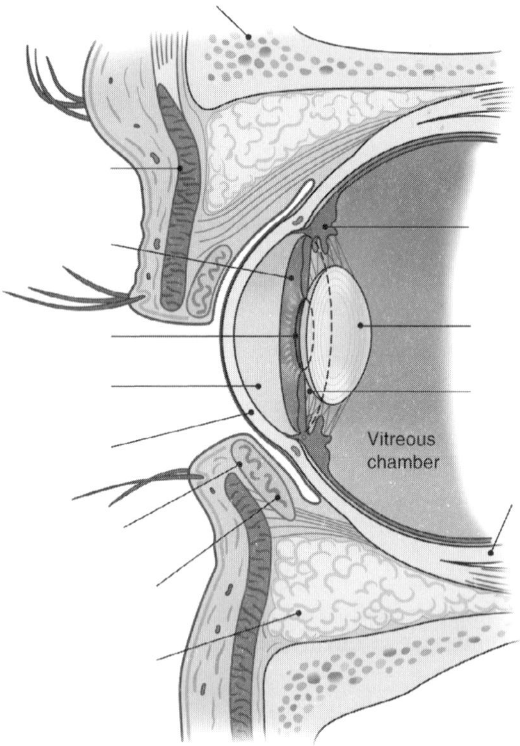

a. Optic disc
b. Physiological cup
c. Macula
d. Fovea centralis
e. Artery
f. Vein

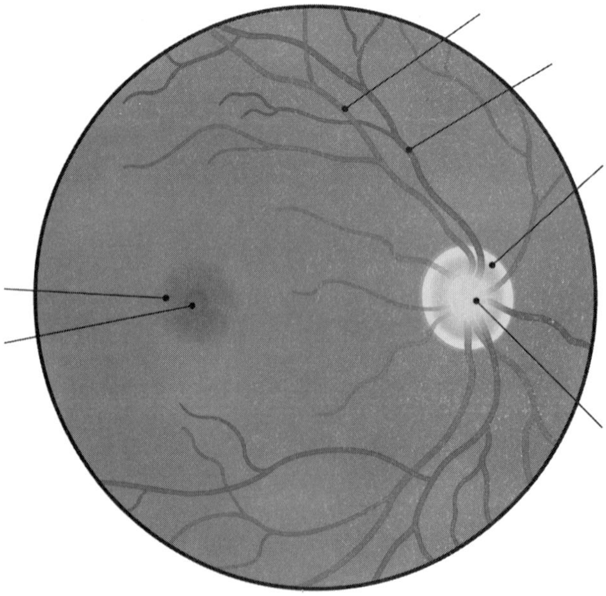

Right eye

2. Match the structures in the first column to their specific functions in the second column.

Structure	Function
1. Bulbar conjunctiva	a. Drain for aqueous humor; helps control intraocular pressure (IOP)
2. Cornea	b. Area of central vision
3. Lens	c. Area where optic nerve enters eye
4. Iris	d. Biconvex disc through which light and images pass
5. Palpebral conjunctiva	e. Colored, circular muscular diaphragm
6. Sclera	f. Mucous membrane that lines eyeball
7. Lacrimal gland	g. Clear, jelly-like substance that cushions retina and helps maintain eye shape
8. Macula	h. Area between cornea and iris
9. Optic disc	i. Area between iris and lens
10. Anterior chamber	j. White, tough avascular layer that gives eye structure and shape
11. Canal of Schlemm	k. Produces tears
12. Posterior chamber	l. Clear fluid that supplies lens and cornea with nutrition
13. Vitreous humor	m. Mucous membrane that lines eyelids
14. Aqueous humor	n. Outer layer of eye; avascular and transparent

3. Dan Jordan, a 55-year-old man with type 2 diabetes, is here for his annual eye exam. When you measure his visual acuity, the results are OD 20/50, OS 20/40, OU 20/40. Mr. Jordan asks you, "What does this mean?" How would you explain these results to him?

____

____

4. Normal far vision for an adult is 20/20. Would you expect a toddler to have 20/20 vision?

____

____

5. Name three tests used to measure the extraocular muscles.

____

6. Match the structures in the first column with possible abnormal assessment findings in the second column.

Structure	Abnormal Findings
1. Lids	a. Ectropion
2. Lashes	b. Arcus senilis
3. Cornea	c. Xanthelasma
4. Bulbar conjunctiva	d. Cataract
5. Lens	e. "Pink eye"
6. Anterior chamber	f. Jaundice
7. Sclera	g. Increased IOP

7. You are performing a funduscopic exam on Mr. Jordan. Identify three key details to remember when using an ophthalmoscope.

____

____

8. Describe the function of the different light apertures of the ophthalmoscope.

    a. Small white light

    b. Large white light

    c. Blue light

    d. Green light

    e. Grid

    f. Slit of white light

9. Although your assessment focuses on the eyes, all systems are related. What assessment findings (subjective or objective) show the relationship between the eyes and other systems?

____

____

Name ______________________ Date ______________

Course ______________ Instructor ______________

Abnormal Case Study: Brenda Williams

Brenda Williams is a 45-year-old, married African American woman and mother of two. A part-time computer analyst, she presents in the ED with complaints of severe eye pain. Because this is an acute problem, you do a focused assessment. Findings suggest primary angle-closure glaucoma.

Health History

CHIEF COMPLAINT:

"I have terrible eye pain."

Symptom Analysis:

P—No precipitating factor and nothing seems to make it better.

Q—"Feels like someone is stabbing my eye."

R—Colored halos around lights, blurred vision, nausea and vomiting.

S—10/10.

T—Acute onset.

Current Health Status:

- Denies history of eye problems; doesn't wear corrective lenses.
- Denies any medical problems.
- Last eye exam 2 years ago.

Physical Assessment

- *Visual acuity:* Unable to test near and far vision because of blurred vision.
- *Peripheral vision:* Field cuts noted in temporal fields.
- *Extraocular movement:* Intact.
- *External structures:* Eyes red, cornea has frosted appearance.
- *Internal structures:* Optic disc cupping

10. Considering Mrs. Williams's diagnosis of primary angle-closure glaucoma, what additional history question should you ask her? Why?

____

11. What additional test is indicated in view of Mrs. Williams's presenting signs and symptoms?

____

12. Primary angle-closure glaucoma is considered a medical ocular emergency. What would likely result if Mrs. Williams's problem goes untreated?

____

13. What factor placed Mrs. Williams at risk for glaucoma?

____

14. Cluster the data for the following nursing diagnoses:

a. Pain related to increased intraocular pressure.

____

____

b. Risk for injury related to visual acuity deficits.

____

____

c. Disturbed sensory perception (vision) related to pathological process.

____

____

15. Identify any additional nursing diagnoses for Mrs. Williams.

____

____

16. *Word jumble:* Unscramble the following words. Then unscramble the circled letters to complete the sentence: Always examine the ________ last on funduscopic exam.

1. L A (C) R S E
2. R S I I
3. A L D E (M) I C U S T H N A
4. E N R C A O
5. L R C I (L) M A A L N D A G
6. T A I N R E
7. (A) N V T I C J N U O C
8. (U) P L I P
9. N S E L
10. E V O F (A)

Name ______________________ Date ______________

Course ______________ Instructor ______________

Student Lab Sheet: Assessing the Eyes

Client's Initials: ______________

Age: ______________

Gender: ______________

Health History

BIOGRAPHICAL DATA:

Current Health Status: Symptom Analysis (PQRST)

- Vision loss
- Tearing
- Eye pain
- Changes in eye appearance
- Blurred vision
- Dry eyes
- Double vision
- Drainage

Past Health History:

- Childhood illnesses
- Hospitalizations
- Surgeries
- Serious injuries/chronic illness
- Immunizations
- Allergies (food, drugs, environmental)
- Medications (prescribed and over-the-counter [OTC])
- Recent travel/military service

Family History:

Review of Systems:

- General health status
- Head, eyes, ears, nose, and throat (HEENT)
- Respiratory
- Cardiovascular
- Gastrointestinal
- Genitourinary
- Musculoskeletal
- Neurologic
- Endocrine
- Lymphatic/hematological

Psychosocial Profile:

- Health practices and beliefs/self-care activities
- Typical day
- Nutritional patterns (24-hour recall)
- Activity/exercise patterns
- Recreation, pets, hobbies
- Sleep/rest patterns
- Personal habits (tobacco, alcohol, caffeine, and drugs)
- Occupational health patterns
- Socioeconomic status
- Environmental health patterns
- Roles, relationships, self-concept
- Cultural/religious influences
- Family roles/relationships
- Sexuality patterns
- Social supports
- Stress/coping

Physical Assessment

GENERAL SURVEY:

- Vital signs
- Height
- Weight

Head-to-Toe Scan:

- Integumentary
- Head, nose, throat
- Respiratory
- Cardiovascular
- Abdomen
- Genitourinary
- Musculoskeletal
- Neurologic

Assessment of the Eyes

Area/Physical Assessment Skill	Assessment	Normal Findings Developmental/Cultural Variations	Student's Findings
Visual acuity	**Measure each eye separately, then together, with and without corrective lenses.** **Tests CN I.**		
Far	Depending on patient's age and literacy level, use Snellen eye chart, Snellen E chart, or Stycar chart. Visual acuity represented by fraction with **numerator 20—number of feet patient stands from chart—and denominator—number of feet someone with 20/20 vision can read chart—e.g., 20/40 vision.** **No more than two mistakes per line.**	20/20 OD, OS, OU Child's vision does not reach 20/20 until around age 6 or 7.	
Near	Assess ability to read newsprint held 13 to 15 inches from eyes. Use print-sized pictures if patient unable to read.	Near vision intact. Presbyopia (farsightedness) commonly occurs with aging.	
Color vision	Differentiate patterns of colors on color plates or identify color bars on Snellen eye chart.	Color vision intact.	
Peripheral vision	Assess ability to detect movement coming in from periphery (inferior, superior, temporal, and nasal fields). ***Sudden loss of peripheral vision may be a sign of acute glaucoma, a medical emergency. Needs immediate ophthalmology referral.***	Peripheral vision intact OU, all fields.	
Extraocular muscles	Inspect eyes for parallel alignment and corneal light reflex **(look for the sparkle in eyes).** Put eyes through range of motion (ROM), six cardinal fields of vision **(tests CN III, IV, VI).** Perform cover-uncover test, check for drifting.	Eyes in parallel alignment. Corneal light reflex symmetrical, extraocular movement intact OU, no lid lag or nystagmus. No wandering with cover-uncover test.	

INSPECTION			
External eye structures	**Position: sitting**		
General appearance	Note appearance and parallel alignment.	Eyes clear and bright. Equal parallel alignment.	
Eyelids	Note color, lesions, edema, lid lag, and symmetry of palpebral fissures **(opening of eyes between upper and lower lids)**.	Color consistent with patient's complexion. No lesions or edema. Palpebral fissures symmetrical. No lid lag.	
Eyelashes	Note symmetry and distribution. Note entropion, ectropion.	Eyelashes evenly distributed, no ectropion or entropion.	
Lacrimal ducts, puncta	Note color, edema, excessive tearing, or drainage.	Puncta pale pink and patent, no excessive tearing or dryness, drainage, or edema.	
Conjunctiva	Assess color, moisture, lesions, and foreign bodies. **Palpebral conjunctiva covers lids; bulbar conjunctiva covers eyeball.**	Conjunctiva clear, pink, and moist; no lesions.	
Sclera	Note color, moisture, and lesions or tears.	Sclera white and intact, no lesions or tears. Brown spots, muddy sclera, may be seen in persons with dark skin.	
Cornea	Examine cornea from oblique angle. Note clarity, lesions, or abrasions. Test corneal reflex (CNs V and VII). **Instead of touching cornea with wisp of cotton, use a needleless syringe and either shoot small amount of air over cornea or gently touch lashes and look for blink reflex.**	Cornea clear without opacities, lesions, or abrasions. Arcus senilis (white ring around the edge of cornea) common finding in elderly. Positive corneal reflex.	
Anterior chamber	Inspect for clarity, bulging of iris, and blood. **To inspect with patient's eyes looking straight ahead, look across eye from the side.**	Anterior chamber clear, no blood or bulging of iris.	
Iris	Note color, size, shape, and symmetry.	Irises round and symmetrical.	

(continued)

Assessment of the Eyes (continued)

Area/Physical Assessment Skill	Assessment	Normal Findings Developmental/Cultural Variations	Student's Findings
Pupils	Note size, shape, reaction to light (direct and consensual), and test for accommodation. **Tests CN III *intracranial pressure.*** **Consensual reaction: Pupil not receiving light stimulus reacts same as pupil receiving stimulus.** ***Changes in pupils, such as unequal or dilated, may be a sign of increased intracranial pressure.***	Pupil size 3 to 5 mm. Normal size depends on age, larger in children, smaller in elderly. No miosis or mydriasis. Pupils equal, round, reactive to light, and accommodation direct and consensual (PERRLA). Reaction to light: pupils constrict. Accommodation: Pupils converge and constrict. Older patient may have decreased accommodation. Anisocoria (unequal pupils) if < 0.5 mm can be normal variation.	
PALPATION	**Maintain standard precautions.** **Wear gloves if there is eye drainage.**		
Eyeball	**Gently palpate globe with fingertips or thumb on upper lids over sclera.** Note consistency and tenderness. ***Do not palpate eyeball in patients with eye trauma or known glaucoma.***	Eyeball firm and nontender.	
Lacrimal apparatus (tear glands and ducts)	Palpate below eyebrow and inner canthus of eye. Note tenderness or excessive tearing or discharge from punctae.	Lacrimal gland nontender, no drainage or excessive tearing.	
OPHTHALMOSCOPY	**Perform in dark room. Examine same eye to same eye (your right eye to patient's right eye). Use small white light for undilated pupil.**		
Red reflex	Note presence, opacities. **Approach from oblique angle, about 14 inches from patient.**	Positive red reflex, no opacities.	

Optic disc and physiological cup	**Located nasally.** Note size, shape, borders, color, cup: disc ratio.	Optic disc round, with sharp margins; cup:disc ratio 1:2 disc diameters (DD). Color depends on patient's pigmentation. Yellow-to-orange with white cup.	
Retinal vessels	Assess size ratio of arteries and veins, color, arteriole light reflex, crossings. **Arteries and veins come out of disc in pairs. Veins normally darker and larger than arteries.**	Vessels noted. Arteriovenous ratio 2:3 or 4:5. Positive arteriole light reflex. Arteriovenous crossings smooth, no nicking or narrowing.	
Retina	Assess color, texture, exudates, lesions, hemorrhages, or aneurysms.	Color varies from pale yellow to orange-red, depending on patient's pigmentation. The darker the person, the darker the background. Texture finely granular. No lesions, hemorrhages, exudates, or aneurysms.	
Macula, fovea centralis	**Always examine last.** Note, color, size, location, and lesions. **Macula is darker area temporal to disc.**	Macula darker area on retina, 2 DD temporal to OD, 1 DD in size, no lesions, and positive fovea light reflex.	

(continued)

Assessment of the Eyes (continued)

Pertinent Health History Findings:

Pertinent Physical Assessment Findings:

Nursing Diagnoses (Actual or Potential) With Clustered Data:

Name		Date	
Course		Instructor	

Self-Evaluation Exercise

Eyes	Yes	No	Needs More Practice
1. Applies knowledge of anatomy and physiology of the eye in performing an eye assessment.			
2. Applies growth and development principles as applicable to the eye.			
3. Considers cultural variations as indicated when performing an eye assessment.			
4. Gathers all equipment necessary to perform an eye assessment.			
5. Obtains history specific to assessment of the eye.			
6. Performs a physical assessment of the eye, including: • General survey and head-to-toe scan. • Visual testing. • Inspection of external structures. • Palpation of external structures. • Ophthalmoscopy.			
7. Documents eye assessment findings.			
8. Identifies normal/abnormal findings.			
9. Clusters pertinent subjective/objective data.			
10. Identifies actual/potential health problems and states them as nursing diagnoses with supporting data.			

Name ______________________________ Date ______________

Course ______________________ Instructor ______________________

The Ear

1. Anatomy review: Label the following ear structures:

   a. Helix

   b. Tragus

   c. Lobule

   d. Antitragus

   e. Antihelix

   f. External auditory canal

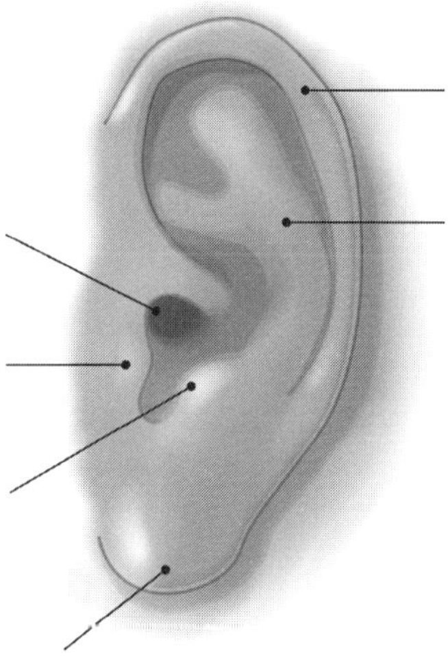

   a. Pars tensa

   b. Pars flaccida

   c. Cone of light

   d. Umbo

   e. Malleus

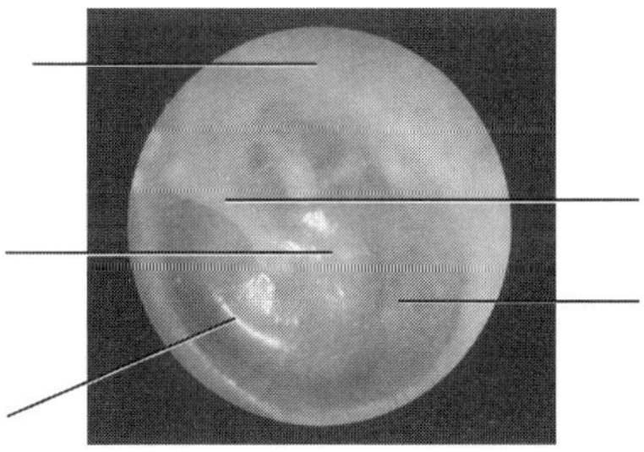

2. Match the structures in the first column to their specific functions in the second column.

Structure	Function
1. Auricle	a. Light reflection on tympanic membrane
2. Tympanic membrane	b. Located in inner ear; organ of hearing that transmits sound to cranial nerve (CN) VIII
3. Cochlea	c. External ear; collects sound waves
4. Auditory ossicles	d. Eardrum
5. Cone of light	e. Tube from middle ear to nasopharynx that equalizes pressure in middle ear
6. Organ of Corti	f. Ear wax
7. Eustachian tube	g. Smallest bones of body in middle ear; transmit sound vibrations
8. Cerumen	h. Shell-like structure in inner ear that transmits sound vibrations

3. Mrs. Hudson says that her son, Jimmy, age 2, has had a fever for 2 days and started complaining of an earache today. Part of your assessment should include examining the ears. You discover that Jimmy's gross hearing is diminished. List five questions that may help you identify contributing/risk factors for hearing loss.

____

____

4. You perform the Weber test on Jimmy, checking for lateralization of sound. If Jimmy had a conductive hearing loss, to which ear would the sound lateralize? If he has a sensorineural hearing loss, to which ear would the sound lateralize?

____

5. Next, you perform the Rinne test to compare bone conduction (BC) with air conduction (AC). What would you expect the normal findings to be? What findings would you expect if Jimmy has a conductive hearing loss?

____

____

6. Now, inspect Jimmy's external ear and look for drainage. Name three types of drainage you might see, and describe the significance of each.

____

____

7. Before you perform the otoscopic exam, name three places that you need to palpate for tenderness before otoscope insertion.

____

____

8. To straighten a young child's ear canal, which way should the auricle be positioned? What about an adult's ear canal?

____

9. Name three characteristics you should note when assessing the tympanic membrane.

____

10. Jimmy's eardrum is red and bulging. Mrs. Hudson says, "Jimmy gets a lot of ear infections. Why?" How would you answer this question?

____

____

11. Although your assessment focuses on the ears, all systems are related. What assessment findings (subjective or objective) show the relationship between the ears and other systems?

____

____

Name ______________________ Date ______________

Course ______________ Instructor ______________

Abnormal Case Study: Brian Chapin

Mrs. Chapin brings her 3-year-old son, Brian, for treatment of recurrent earache. Brian has had frequent ear infections. He caught a cold last week and now is irritable, tugging at his ear, and not sleeping or eating well. His temperature is 101°F.

Health History

CHIEF COMPLAINT:

"My ear hurts."

Current Health Status:

- Recent upper respiratory infection.
- Mother reports irritability, tugging at ear, not sleeping or eating well.
- History of recurrent ear infections.
- No known allergies to drugs, food, or environmental factors.
- Family history of otitis media; father had frequent ear infections as a child.

Physical Assessment

- Tugging at ear and irritable.
- Temperature 101°F.
- External ear tenderness.
- External ear canal patent, no drainage.
- Tympanic membrane red and bulging, diffuse cone of light, no perforation.
- Productive cough, yellow mucus.
- Red pharynx.
- Tonsils enlarged and red without exudates.
- Lungs clear.

12. What factors put Brian at risk for otitis media?

____

____

13. What other history findings would identify additional risk factors for otitis media?

____

14. Considering Brian's findings, what additional assessment of the tympanic membrane is indicated?

____

15. Cluster the supporting data for the following nursing diagnoses:

    a. Pain related to increased fluid and pressure in the ear.

    ____

    ____

    b. Risk for disturbed sensory perception (hearing) related to pathological process.

    ____

    ____

    c. Risk for fluid volume deficit.

    ____

    ____

    d. Sleep pattern disturbance.

    ____

16. Identify any additional nursing diagnoses for Brian.

    ____

    ____

17. *Word jumble:* Unscramble the following words. Then unscramble the circled letters to complete the sentence: Another word for swimmer's ear is __________.

    1. T S I O I T (E) D I M A
    2. G T U S A (R)
    3. O S T M D A (I)
    4. C S I (N) U
    5. L O L M U A S (E) L
    6. E P S (A) T S
    7. H C E A L (O) C
    8. I H (L) E (X)
    9. S (I) X (S) O E (T) I O S
    10. A L C O H M (T) E S E O A T

Name ______________________________ Date ______________

Course ______________________ Instructor ______________________

Student Lab Sheet: Assessing the Ears

Client's Initials: ______________________

Age: ______________________

Gender: ______________________

Health History

BIOGRAPHICAL DATA:

Current Health Status:
Symptom Analysis (PQRST):

- Hearing loss
- Vertigo
- Tinnitus
- Otorrhea
- Otalgia

Past Health History:

- Childhood illnesses
- Hospitalizations
- Surgeries
- Serious injuries/chronic illness
- Immunizations
- Allergies (food, drugs, environmental)
- Medications (prescribed and OTC)
- Recent travel/military service

Family History:

Review of Systems:

- General health status
- Head, nose, throat
- Respiratory
- Cardiovascular
- Gastrointestinal
- Genitourinary
- Musculoskeletal
- Neurologic
- Endocrine
- Lymphatic/hematological

Psychosocial Profile:

- Health practices and beliefs/self-care activities
- Typical day
- Nutritional patterns (24-hour recall)
- Activity/exercise patterns
- Recreation, pets, hobbies
- Sleep/rest patterns
- Personal habits (tobacco, alcohol, caffeine, and drugs)
- Occupational health patterns
- Socioeconomic status
- Environmental health patterns
- Roles, relationships, self-concept
- Cultural/religious influences
- Family roles/relationships
- Sexuality patterns
- Social supports
- Stress/coping

Physical Assessment

GENERAL SURVEY:

- Vital signs
- Height
- Weight

Head-to-Toe Scan:

- Integumentary
- Head, nose, throat
- Respiratory
- Cardiovascular
- Abdomen
- Genitourinary
- Musculoskeletal
- Neurologic

Assessment of Ears

Area/Physical Assessment Skill	Assessment	Normal Findings Developmental/Cultural Variations	Student's Findings
INSPECTION	**Position: Sitting; supine for infant to immobilize head.**		
External ear	Note position, shape, size, symmetry, color, lesions, and drainage (clear, bloody, or purulent). ***Clear drainage from nose or ears, secondary to head trauma may be cerebrospinal fluid (CSF).*** Note angle of attachment **(draw imaginary line from top of helix to external canthus of eye, then a perpendicular line in front of ear).**	Vertical ear position with $<$ 10 degree lateral posterior slant. Ears aligned with eyes, symmetrical, no redness, lesions, or drainage.	
PALPATION	**Maintain standard precautions.** **Wear gloves if drainage present.**		
External ear	Assess consistency, tenderness, and lesions. **Palpate tragus and mastoid process, and pull helix forward before inserting otoscope. Tenderness may signal ear infection, so proceed carefully.**	Helix soft and pliable, nontender, no nodules or lesions.	
OTOSCOPIC EXAM	**Use largest and shortest speculum ear canal can accommodate (4, 5, or 6 mm, 0.5 inch). Have patient tilt head to opposite side being examined.** **Pull helix up and back for adult and down for child. Always look into canal before inserting otoscope.** **Insert 0.5 inch for an adult; insert 0.25 inch for child. Avoid inner two-thirds of canal, which is over temporal bone and is sensitive.** Note color, drainage, patency, edema, lesions, or foreign objects. **Cerumen is only normal drainage in ear.**		

External ear canal	Note position of landmarks (cone of light, pars flaccida, pars tensa, malleus, and umbo). **Ears are mirror images, cone of light is at 7 o'clock in left ear and 5 o'clock in right ear.**	Ear canal light colored and patent; small amount of yellow cerumen and hair; no lesions, exudates, or foreign objects. Color and amount of cerumen varies depending on ethnicity.	
Tympanic membrane	Note intactness of tympanic membrane, color, lesions, and exudates. Assess mobility of tympanic membrane in children. Use pneumatic attachment to assess mobility of tympanic membrane. ***Never irrigate ear canal unless you are sure tympanic membrane is intact.***	Tympanic membrane pearly gray, intact, mobile, no lesions or exudates. Landmarks appropriately noted. No bulging or retraction of tympanic membrane.	
HEARING	**Test each ear separately.**		
Gross hearing	Whispered voice test to assess for low-pitched deficits **(1 to 2 feet from ear).** Ticking watch test to assess for high-pitch deficits **(5 inches from ear).**	Gross hearing intact bilaterally.	
Weber test	Place vibrating tuning fork on forehead or top of head to assess BC. **Do not touch prongs of tuning fork—It dampens vibration.**	Negative lateralization of sound, heard equally in both ears.	
Rinne test	Compare BC with AC. Place vibrating tuning fork on mastoid (BC) until no longer heard, then move fork to in front of ear (AC). Time how long sound is heard.	Sound transmission through air is normally twice as long as sound transmission through bone. AC > BC.	
BALANCE			
Romberg test	Perform Romberg test (see Chapter 20 Assessing the Motor-Musculoskeletal System) with eyes open, then closed.	Negative Romberg.	

(continued)

Assessment of Ears (continued)

Pertinent Health History Findings:

Pertinent Physical Assessment Findings:

Nursing Diagnoses (Actual or Potential) With Clustered Data:

Name ______________________________ Date ______________

Course ______________________ Instructor ______________________

Self-Evaluation Exercise

Ear	Yes	No	Needs More Practice
1. Applies knowledge of anatomy and physiology of the ear in performing an ear assessment.			
2. Applies growth and development principles as applicable to the ear.			
3. Considers cultural variations as indicated when performing an ear assessment.			
4. Gathers all equipment necessary to perform an ear assessment.			
5. Obtains history specific to assessment of the ear.			
6. Performs a physical assessment of the ear, including: • General survey and head-to-toe scan. • Hearing testing. • Inspection of external structures. • Palpation of external structures. • Otoscopic exam.			
7. Documents ear assessment findings.			
8. Identifies normal/abnormal findings.			
9. Clusters pertinent subjective/objective data.			
10. Identifies actual/potential health problems and states them as nursing diagnoses with supporting data.			

Chapter 13

Assessing the Respiratory System

Name		Date	
Course		Instructor	

1. Anatomy review: Label the following structures.
   a. Nasal cavity
   b. Nasopharynx
   c. Oropharynx
   d. Laryngopharynx
   e. Esophagus
   f. Trachea
   g. Larynx
   h. Right bronchial tree
   i. Left bronchial tree
   j. Mediastinum
   k. Parietal pleura
   l. Pulmonary artery
   m. Terminal bronchiole
   n. Capillaries
   o. Pulmonary vein
   p. Alveolar duct
   q. Alveolus
   r. Interalveolar septum
   s. Acinus

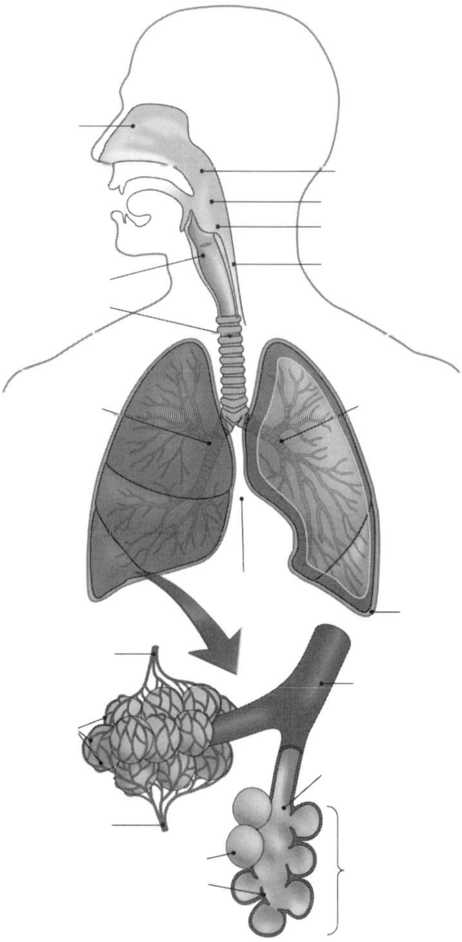

2. Match the structures in the first column to their specific functions in the second column.

Structure	Function
1. Nasal cavity	a. Prevents food from entering trachea
2. Pleura	b. Primary muscle for breathing
3. Alveoli	c. Warms and filters air
4. Diaphragm	d. Contains vocal cords
5. Epiglottis	e. Protective lining of lung
6. Larynx	f. Functional unit of lung

3. Match the respiratory sounds in the first column to the descriptions in the second column.

Breath Sound	Description
1. Vesicular	a. Abnormal voice sound "ee" to "aa"
2. Crackles	b. High-pitched musical sound heard during acute asthmatic attack
3. Bronchial	c. Normal breath sound heard over manubrium with equal respiratory phases
4. Rhonchi	d. "Popping" sound heard predominantly during inspiration; sign of congestive heart failure
5. Bronchovesicular	e. High-pitched inspiratory sound; sign of upper airway obstruction
6. Wheezes	f. Abnormal voice sound, clearer transmission of spoken voice sound
7. Egophony	g. "Rattle" sound primarily heard on expiration in upper airway resulting from secretions
8. Stridor	h. Abnormal voice sound, clearer transmission of whispered voice sound
9. Whispered pectoriloquy	i. Normal breath sound, with inspiration less than expiration; heard over trachea
10. Bronchophony	j. Normal breath sound with inspiration greater than expiration; heard in most lung fields

4. Mabel Terranova, age 78, is admitted to your unit with a diagnosis of aspiration pneumonia of the right middle lobe. She has a history of stroke and difficulty swallowing. While eating lunch, she began to choke and have respiratory difficulty. Considering Mrs. Terranova's age, what normal differences might you expect to find when assessing her respiratory system?

____

____

5. Mrs. Terranova's extremities are pale and dusky. How would you differentiate central cyanosis from peripheral cyanosis?

____

____

6. Cyanotic color changes are a late sign of hypoxia. What physical findings would reflect early hypoxia?

____

____

7. Considering Mrs. Terranova's diagnosis of right middle lobe pneumonia, what sounds might you expect to hear when you auscultate her lungs?

____

____

8. On auscultation, you find that Mrs. Terranova's lungs are clear posteriorly. Considering that she has right middle lobe pneumonia, how do you explain these findings?

____

____

9. On admission, Mrs. Terranova's pulse oxygen level is 87 percent on room air (normal pulse oximetry is 100 percent). Because her oxygen level is low, what changes might you find in her neurologic system, integumentary system, and cardiovascular system?

____

____

____

10. Although your assessment focuses on the respiratory system, all systems are related. What assessment findings (subjective or objective) show the relationship between the respiratory system and other systems?

____

____

____

Name ______________________ Date ______________

Course ______________ Instructor ______________

Abnormal Case Study: Raymond Augustus

Raymond Augustus, a 65-year-old African American man, is admitted to the respiratory unit with exacerbation of emphysema. He has had the disease for 10 years and is well known to the staff, having been in and out of the hospital several times. Recently, his hospitalizations have become more frequent. A frail, thin man on oxygen, he is obviously short of breath at rest with pursed-lip breathing. His wife, who accompanies him, comments, "Here we go again!" You take him to his room and make him as comfortable as possible before beginning his admission assessment. Because Mr. Augustus is in mild respiratory distress, you postpone taking a complete history and focus on his chief complaint.

Health History

CHIEF COMPLAINT:

"I can't get my breath and I have a cough."

Symptom Analysis:

P—Increased shortness of breath; breathes better when sitting.

Q—Feels like "I can't get enough air."

R—"It's my breathing; my chest is sore from coughing, and I'm so tired."

S—On a scale from 1 to 10, with 10 being the worst, how disabling is this problem? +10

T—Diagnosed with emphysema 10 years ago, has gotten progressively worse to point where he has shortness of breath at rest.

Current Health History:

Shortness of breath when performing activities of daily living (ADL) (grade 3). You compare this with the patient's last admission 7 months ago and see that at that time he had shortness of breath with mild activity (grade 2). This helps you determine progression of disease and its effect on the patient's life.

- Dyspnea on exertion and orthopnea. Patient uses four pillows at night to sleep.
- Productive cough with a large amount of thick, foul-smelling, yellow sputum. Cough sounds congested and had acute onset. *Note:* Mr. Augustus has emphysema; he is not a mucus producer.
- Weight gain of 5 lb in past week; feet are also swollen.
- Before onset of productive cough, patient's three grandchildren had visited, and two had colds.
- Patient's chest is sore from coughing, and he complains of fatigue.

11. Based on this information, what do you think triggered this current exacerbation?

____

____

12. What do you think caused the 5-lb weight gain and swollen feet?

____

____

Complete Health History:

When the patient's condition stabilizes, proceed with a complete health history.

Past Health History:

- Multiple admissions over past 10 years for emphysema.
- Received flu shot in October of this year.
- Current medications include a bronchodilator, diuretic, potassium supplement, and "heart pill."

Family History:

- Father had emphysema.

Psychosocial Profile:

- *Nutritional patterns:* Poor appetite because eating tires him and he becomes short of breath.
- *Recreation/hobbies:* Loves to fish, but this is becoming more difficult because of illness.
- *Occupational health patterns:* Patient was a truck driver forced into early retirement because of emphysema. He experienced possible exposure to air pollutants secondary to job.
- *Environmental health patterns:* Lives in city in a two-story duplex with hot-air heat and no central air conditioning. May be exposed to air pollutants secondary to urban residence and home heating system.
- *Roles/relationships:* Lives with wife of 45 years, who is primary support person and caregiver. They rarely socialize with friends and family because of his medical problems and have not been sexually active for some time because of his fatigue and breathing difficulties.

Physical Assessment

- *General appearance:* Appears older than stated age of 65 years; frail; facial expression tired and slightly anxious; position of comfort—tripod.
- *Vital signs:* Temperature 100.2°F; pulse 98 beats per minute (BPM), regular; respirations 28/min, shallow with effort and prolonged expiratory phase; blood pressure (BP) 150/94 mm Hg; weight 115 lb (underweight); height 5 feet, 7 inches.
- *Inspection:*
  - *Mental status:* Awake, alert, and oriented x 4 (person, place, time, situation); fatigue.
  - *Integumentary:* Skin gray-brown; mucous membranes pale and gray.
  - *Head, eyes, ears, nose, and throat (HEENT):* Trachea midline; positive pursed-lip breathing, neck vein distension, and hypertrophy of neck muscles.
  - *Chest:* Anteroposterior:lateral 1:1, barrel chest; costal angle > 90 degrees; symmetrical rise and fall of chest, but decreased excursion at bases; positive use of accessory muscles; skin intact; prominent ribs and intercostals, but no retraction; no spinal deformities.
  - *Extremities:* Capillary refill > 6 seconds; positive clubbing; nail beds pale and gray; pedal edema.
- *Palpation:*
  - Trachea midline.
  - Chest nontender.
  - Decreased excursion at bases.
  - Increased tactile fremitus over upper lobes.
- *Percussion:*
  - Level of diaphragm T12 posterior.
  - Hyperresonance at bases; dullness over upper lobes.
  - Diaphragmatic excursion: no change between inspiration and expiration.
- *Auscultation:*
  - Decreased breath sounds at bases.
  - Scattered rhonchi and expiratory wheezes throughout lung fields.

13. What signs/symptoms would you expect to see in a patient with nail clubbing?

____

____

14. How would you explain the fact that Mr. Augustus's diaphragm is at T12 level with no change in diaphragmatic excursion?

____

____

15. What assessment findings are consistent with Mr. Augustus's diagnosis of emphysema?

____

____

16. Cluster the supporting data for the following nursing diagnoses:

    a. Ineffective airway clearance related to increased secretions and fatigue.

    ____

    ____

    b. Impaired gas exchange related to alveoli destruction.

    ____

    ____

    c. Nutrition less than body requirements related to dyspnea.

    ____

    ____

17. Identify any additional nursing diagnoses for Mr. Augustus.

____

____

18. *Word search:* Find the following words in the puzzle: alveoli, asthma, bronchial, egophony, lobe, lung, trachea, vesicular, wheeze.

Y	Y	N	O	H	P	O	L	B	Y
L	L	O	B	E	B	W	H	I	Y
W	U	T	R	A	C	H	E	A	N
I	N	E	O	P	W	E	E	R	O
E	G	O	N	P	H	E	E	A	H
U	L	U	C	G	E	Z	Z	C	P
E	V	W	H	E	E	Z	E	H	O
V	E	S	I	C	U	L	A	R	G
U	T	R	A	S	T	H	M	A	E
A	S	A	L	V	E	O	L	I	B

Name ______________________ Date ______________

Course ______________ Instructor ______________

Student Lab Sheet: Assessing the Respiratory System

Client's Initials: ______________

Age: ______________

Gender: ______________

Health History

BIOGRAPHICAL DATA:

Current Health Status: Symptom Analysis (PQRST):

- Cough
- Dyspnea (difficulty breathing, shortness of breath)
- Chest pain
- Related symptoms (edema and fatigue)

Past Health History:

- Childhood illnesses
- Hospitalizations
- Surgeries
- Serious injuries/chronic illness
- Immunizations
- Allergies (food, drugs, environmental)
- Medications (prescribed and over-the-counter [OTC])
- Recent travel/military service

Family History:

Review of Systems:

- General health status
- HEENT
- Cardiovascular
- Gastrointestinal
- Genitourinary
- Musculoskeletal
- Neurologic
- Endocrine
- Lymphatic/hematological

Psychosocial Profile:

- Health practices and beliefs/self-care activities
- Typical day
- Nutritional patterns (24-hour recall)
- Activity/exercise patterns
- Recreation, pets, hobbies
- Sleep/rest patterns
- Personal habits (tobacco, alcohol, caffeine, and drugs)
- Occupational health patterns
- Socioeconomic status
- Environmental health patterns
- Roles, relationships, self-concept
- Cultural/religious influences
- Family roles/relationships
- Sexuality patterns
- Social supports
- Stress/coping

Physical Assessment

GENERAL SURVEY:

- Vital signs
- Height
- Weight

Head-to-Toe Scan:

- General health status
- Integumentary
- HEENT
- Cardiovascular
- Abdomen
- Genitourinary
- Musculoskeletal
- Neurologic

Assessing the Respiratory System

Area/Physical Assessment Skill	Assessment	Normal Findings Developmental/Cultural Variations	Student's Findings
INSPECTION	**Anterior/posterior/lateral. Compare side to side, work apex to base.** **Position: Sitting.**		
Chest	Assess respiratory rate, rhythm, depth, symmetry of chest movements. Assess anteroposterior:lateral ratio, costal angle, spinal deformities, muscles for breathing, and condition of skin.	Respiratory rate varies with age. Respirations quiet, symmetrical, with regular rhythm and depth. Anteroposterior:lateral ratio 1:2, costal angle < 90 degrees, no barrel chest or spinal deformities. No retraction or use of accessory muscles, skin intact. Senile emphysema, increased. Anteroposterior:lateral ratio 1.1 may be seen in older patients. Costal angle increases during pregnancy. Women are more thoracic breathers; men and infants are more abdominal breathers.	
PALPATION	**Anterior/posterior/lateral.** **Compare side to side, apex to base.**		
Trachea	Place fingers on either side of trachea to assess position.	Trachea midline, no deviation.	
Chest	Assess for chest tenderness, masses, crepitus. Assess excursion at bases if abnormal, assess apices. Assess tactile fremitus, estimate level of diaphragm, note increased or decreased areas of fremitus. **Use balls or ulnar surface of your hands; have patient say "99."**	Chest nontender, no masses or crepitus. Symmetrical excursion anteriorly and posteriorly. No lags. Tactile fremitus equal bilaterally, anteriorly, and posteriorly.	
PERCUSSION	**Use indirect (mediate) percussion.** **Anterior/posterior/lateral.** **Compare side to side, apex to base.**		

Chest	Note general percussion sound of chest. To assess diaphragmatic excursion, percuss level of diaphragm on full expiration and full inspiration, then measure.	*Anterior chest:* Resonance to second intercostal space (ICS) on the left, to fourth ICS on right. *Lateral chest:* Resonance to eighth ICS. *Posterior chest:* Resonance to T10, and T12 on inspiration. Diaphragmatic excursion 3 to 6 cm bilaterally.	
AUSCULTATION	**Use diaphragm of stethoscope. Have patient take slow, deep breaths through mouth.** **Anterior/posterior/lateral.** **Compare side to side, apex to base.**		
Breath sounds	**Listen through one full respiratory cycle at each site.** Assess normal breath sounds, abnormal sounds, and adventitious sounds (crackles, rhonchi, wheezes, pleural friction rub). Assess for abnormal voice sounds if indicated. **Note relationship of inspiration to expiration, pitch, intensity, and location of sounds.**	All lungs fields clear to auscultation. Bronchial breath sounds heard over trachea. Bronchovesicular breath sounds heard over manubrium/sternum anteriorly and between scapula posteriorly. Vesicular sounds heard in most lung fields. No abnormal or adventitious breath sounds. No abnormal voice sounds, egophony, bronchophony, or whispered pectoriloquy.	

(continued)

Assessing the Respiratory System (continued)

Pertinent Health History Findings:

Pertinent Physical Assessment Findings:

Nursing Diagnoses (Actual or Potential) With Clustered Data:

Name ______________________________	Date ______________
Course ______________________ Instructor	______________________

Self-Evaluation Exercise

Respiratory System	Yes	No	Needs More Practice
1. Applies knowledge of the respiratory system anatomy and physiology in performing a respiratory assessment.			
2. Applies growth and development principles as applicable to the respiratory system.			
3. Considers cultural variations as indicated when performing a respiratory assessment.			
4. Gathers all equipment necessary to perform a respiratory assessment.			
5. Obtains history specific to assessment of the respiratory system.			
6. Performs a physical assessment of the respiratory system, including: • General survey and head-to-toe scan. • Inspection. • Palpation. • Percussion. • Auscultation.			
7. Documents respiratory assessment findings.			
8. Identifies normal/abnormal findings.			
9. Clusters pertinent subjective/objective data.			
10. Identifies actual/potential health problems and states them as nursing diagnoses with supporting data.			

Chapter 14

Assessing the Cardiovascular System

Name ______________________ Date ______________

Course ______________ Instructor ______________________

1. Anatomy review: Label the following structures:
   a. Right atrium
   b. Right ventricle
   c. Right pulmonary arteries
   d. Right pulmonary veins
   e. Mitral (atrioventricular [AV]) valve
   f. Aortic arch
   g. Aortic semilunar valve
   h. Pulmonary semilunar valve
   i. Thoracic aorta
   j. Inferior vena cava
   k. Interventricular septum
   l. Myocardium
   m. Epicardium
   n. Tricuspid (AV) valve
   o. Superior vena cava
   p. Subepicardial fat and connective tissue
   q. Fibrous pericardium
   r. Coronary artery and vein
   s. Epicardium or visceral pericardium
   t. Serous pericardium parietal layer
   u. Left atrium
   v. Left ventricle
   w. Left pulmonary artery
   x. Left pulmonary veins
   y. Pericardium
   z. Pericardial space
   zz. Endocardium

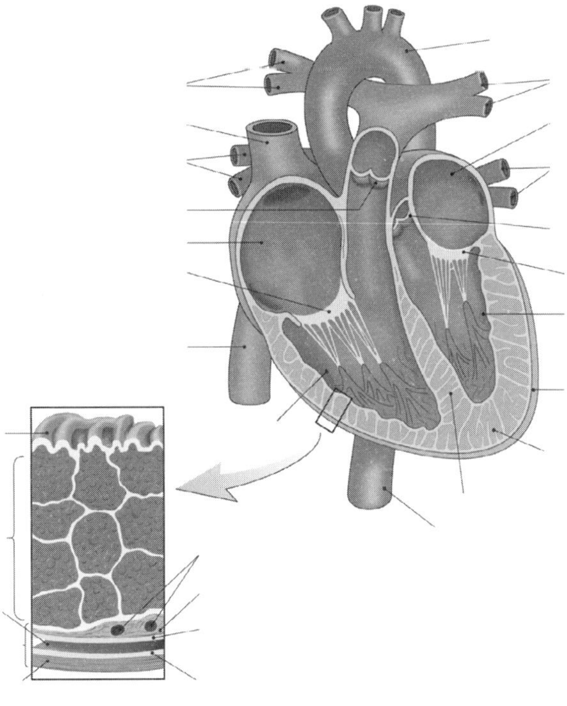

a. AV node
b. Superior vena cava
c. Sinoatrial node
d. Purkinje fibers
e. Left atrium
f. Right atrium
g. AV bundle (bundle of His)
h. Right ventricle
i. Left ventricle
j. Myocardium
k. Left bundle branch
l. Right bundle branch
m. Bachmann's bundle

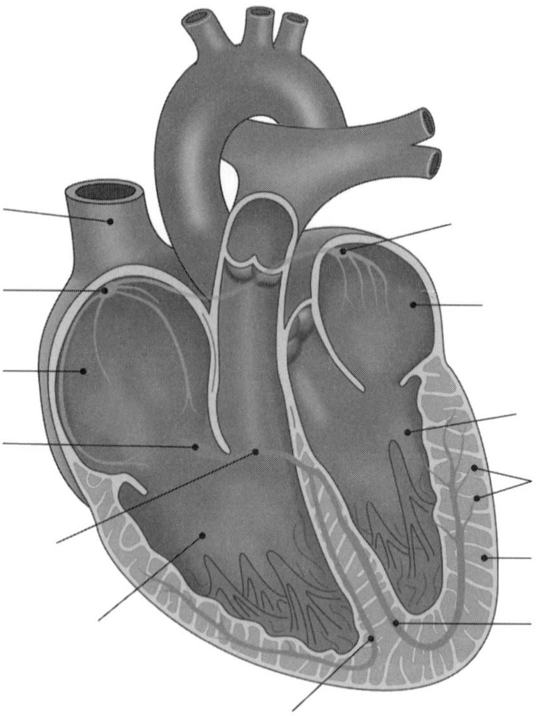

a. Left base
b. Apex
c. Left lateral sternal border (LLSB)
d. Erb's point
e. Right base
f. Aortic valve
g. Mitral valve
h. Tricuspid valve
i. Xiphoid
j. Pulmonic valve

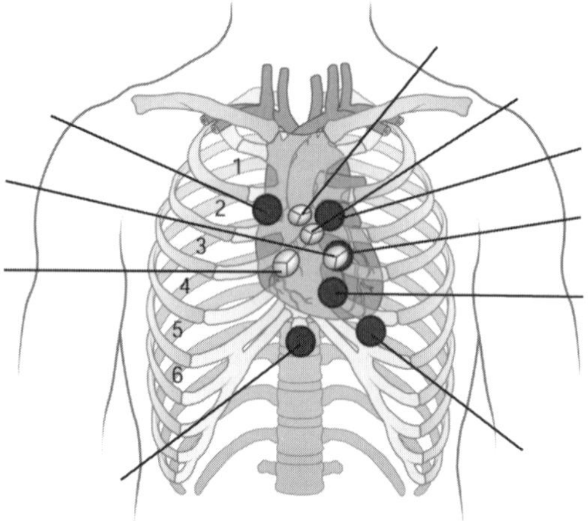

2. Match the structures in the first column to their descriptions in the second column.

Structure	Description
1. Myocardium	a. Valve between right atrium and right ventricle
2. Endocardium	b. Pacemaker of heart at rate of 60 to 100 beats per minute (BPM)
3. Pericardial space	c. Pumps blood to the systemic circulation
4. Right atrium	d. Paces heart at 40 to 60 BPM
5. Left atrium	e. Space between parietal and visceral layer
6. Sinoatrial node	f. Muscle layer of heart
7. Right ventricle	g. Smooth inner layer of heart
8. Left ventricle	h. Pumps blood to pulmonary circulation

9. Tricuspid valve	i. Major vein of head
10. Jugular	j. Major artery that provides blood supply to head
11. Aortic valve	k. Valve between right ventricle and pulmonary artery
12. Mitral valve	l. Valve between left ventricle and aorta
13. Carotid artery	m. Receives oxygenated blood from pulmonary veins
14. Pulmonic valve	n. Valve between left atrium and left ventricle
15. AV node	o. Receives blood from superior and inferior vena cavae

3. Match the heart sounds in the first column to their descriptions in the second column.

Heart Sound	**Description**
1. S_1	a. S_1, S_2, S_3, S_4
2. S_2	b. High-pitched systolic sound occurring when aortic or pulmonic valves open; associated with mitral valve prolapse
3. S_3	c. High-pitched sound occurring when mitral and tricuspid valves close
4. S_4	d. Sound created by turbulent flow
5. Ejection click	e. Each component of S_1 is heard
6. Opening snap	f. Each component of S_2 is heard
7. Split S_1	g. High-pitched sound occurring when aortic and pulmonic valves close
8. Split S_2	h. Low-pitched early diastolic sound that is sign of "distressed" heart; heard with congestive heart failure
9. Murmur	i. Low-pitched late diastolic sound that is sign of "stressed" heart; often heard with hypertension (HTN)
10. Quadruple rhythm	j. High pitched diastolic sound occurring when mitral or tricuspid valves open

4. When auscultating at the apex, which heart sound is normally louder, S_1 or S_2? Which sound is louder when auscultating at the base?

____

____

5. You know that S_1 and S_2 can split. At what site would you expect to hear a normal split S_1? A split S_2?

____

____

6. A split S_2 is often easier to detect than a split S_1 because of a respiratory variation. What effects do respirations have on S_2?

____

____

7. Robert Simons, age 55, presents in the ED with a chief complaint of chest pain. On admission, his vital signs are blood pressure (BP) 170/118 mm Hg; pulse 123 BPM, regular; respirations 24/min. His skin is gray, diaphoretic, and cool. The cardiac monitor shows sinus tachycardia with elevated ST waves. Mr. Simons is started on a nitroglycerin drip. With tachycardia, it is difficult to differentiate S_1 from S_2. Name three ways to establish the timing of the cardiac cycle to differentiate the heart sounds.

8. Mr. Simons also has a history of HTN. Considering his history of HTN and his possible myocardial infarction, what additional heart sound might you expect to hear and why?

9. Mr. Simons develops congestive heart failure. What additional heart sound might you hear and why?

10. You assess Mr. Simons's jugular venous pressure. There are four ways to differentiate the venous pulsation from the carotid pulsation. What are they?

11. What two points are used to measure jugular venous pressure?

12. Establishing timing in the cardiac cycle is essential in identifying heart sounds. Describe how you would differentiate the following sounds. Include the timing of the sound in the cardiac cycle, whether the sound is systolic or diastolic, the area where the sound is heard best, and the pitch of the sound (high or low).

    a. A split S_1 from an S_4.

    b. A split S_1 from an ejection click.

    c. A split S_2 from an S_3.

    d. A split S_3 from an opening snap.

13. Mr. Simons is admitted to the cardiac care unit until his condition stabilizes. On his 3rd postinfarction day, he develops pericarditis. What additional heart sound would you expect to hear? Describe the sound, and identify the site where you would expect to hear it.

____

____

14. Karen Kelly is a 35-year-old woman with a history of mitral valve prolapse. On examination, you detect a murmur. Name five causes of murmurs.

____

____

15. List five characteristics used to describe a murmur.

____

____

16. A murmur may be innocent or indicate pathology. Name two characteristics of murmurs that indicate pathology.

____

____

17. Part of the vascular exam includes auscultation for carotid bruits. When auscultating, what instructions should you give the patient? What part of the stethoscope is best for detecting bruits?

____

____

18. Although your assessment focuses on the cardiovascular system, all systems are related. What assessment findings (subjective or objective) show the relationship between the cardiovascular system and other systems?

____

____

Name ______________________________ Date ______________

Course ______________________ Instructor ______________________

Abnormal Case Study: Henry Brusca

Henry Brusca, a 72-year-old white man, presents in the ED complaining of chest discomfort. He says it started 2 hours ago, after he finished dinner and then awakened from a nap. Mr. Brusca is well known to you. He has been treated for HTN for the past 4 years. In the ED, he is given aspirin and started on a nitroglycerin drip. An electrocardiogram (ECG) and serum cardiac enzyme test are obtained. Mr. Brusca is admitted to the cardiac care unit with the diagnosis of anterior wall myocardial infarction. He asks you, "Am I going to die?" His condition is critical, so you obtain a focused history.

Health History

CHIEF COMPLAINT:

"I have terrible chest pain."

Symptom Analysis:

P—Discomfort started after eating dinner; pain woke him up from a nap; had large meal. States, "I thought it was indigestion, so took some antacids, but nothing seemed to make it better."

Q—"Feels like someone sitting on my chest—pressure!"

R—"Right here in the middle on my chest." No radiation; shortness of breath at rest.

S—10/10.

T—"It started about 0.5 hour after dinner. I never had indigestion this bad before."

Complete Health History

When the patient's condition stabilizes, proceed with the complete health history.

Biographical Data:

- A 72-year-old white man, married, father of seven grown children.
- Self-employed entrepreneur; BS degree in engineering.
- Born and raised in the United States, Italian descent, Catholic religion.
- Blue Cross/Blue Shield medical insurance plan.
- Referral: Follow-up by primary care physician.
- Source: Self, reliable.

Past Health History:

- Previous ECG revealed left ventricular hypertrophy.
- Hospitalized for HTN.
- No known food, drug, or environmental allergies.
- No other previous medical problem.
- No prescribed medications except enalapril (Vasotec), 5 mg twice a day (took today's dose), and weekly use of antacid for indigestion.

Family History:

- Positive family history of HTN, myocardial infarction, and stroke.

Physical Assessment

- *General appearance:* Well-developed, well-groomed 72-year-old white man, in obvious discomfort. Sitting upright clutching chest. Alert and responsive, oriented x 4, affect anxious.
- *Vital signs:* Temperature 100°F; pulse 115 BPM, strong with occasional extra beat; respirations 28/min, shallow; BP 170/105 mm Hg; height 6 feet; weight 275 lb.
- *Integumentary:* Skin intact, pale/ashen, diaphoretic, good turgor; mucous membranes pale gray and moist; poor capillary refill, negative clubbing; skin cool, pale, shiny, and hairless on lower extremities.
- *Head, eyes, ears, nose, and throat (HEENT):* Eyes: Negative periorbital edema; positive arcus

senilis; funduscopic, positive AV knicking and cotton wool; negative papilledema and hemorrhages. Thyroid not palpable.

- *Respiratory:* Lungs: bibasilar crackles, decreased breath sounds at bases because of guarded respirations; anteroposterior:lateral ratio 1:2.
- *Peripheral-vascular:* +1 peripheral pulses.
- *Gastrointestinal:* Abdomen large, round, soft, nontender; positive bowel sounds; negative hepatomegaly; positive pulsation in epigastric area; negative bruits or thrills.
- *Musculoskeletal/neurologic:* Sensory intact, +2 deep tendon reflexes (DTRs), muscle strength equal, positive hand grip, lower extremities +4/5 muscle strength.

FOCUSED PHYSICAL ASSESSMENT FINDINGS

Neck Vessels:

- Positive carotid pulsation, +2; symmetrical with smooth, sharp upstroke and rapid descent; artery stiff; negative for thrills and bruits.
- Neck vein distension, jugular venous pressure at 30 degrees > 3 cm, positive abdominal jugular reflux.

Precordium:

- Positive sustained pulsations displaced lateral to apex, point of maximum impulse (PMI) 3 cm with increased amplitude.
- Slight pulsations also appreciated at LLSB and base, but not as pronounced.
- Negative thrills; cardiac borders percussed third, fourth, and fifth intercostal space (ICS) to the left of the midclavicular line.
- Heart sounds appreciated with tachycardia and irregular rhythm at apex $S_1 > S_2$ and $S_1 < S_2$ at base; positive S_3 and S_4.
- S_2 negative split, at base left $S_1 < S_2$ negative split, at base right $S_1 < S_2$ with an accentuated S_2; negative for murmurs and rubs.

19. What areas are of major concern and warrant continued assessment?

___

20. The PMI is enlarged. What factors may account for this finding?

___

21. Mr. Brusca's physical findings also reveal neck vein distension and an elevated jugular venous pressure. How would you explain these findings?

___

22. How would you explain the presence of an S_3 and S_4 on physical exam?

___

23. Cluster the data for the following nursing diagnoses:

    a. Pain related to tissue ischemia.

    ___

    ___

    b. Anxiety related to threat of dying.

    ___

    ___

c. Ineffective tissue perfusion related to decreased blood flow.

____

____

d. Decreased cardiac output related to altered myocardial contractility.

____

____

24. Which of the above-listed diagnoses would be of highest priority? Why?

____

____

25. Identify any additional nursing diagnoses for Mr. Brusca.

____

____

26. *Word search:* Find the following words in the puzzle: aorta, artery, bruit, carotid, heart, heave, mitral, murmur, vein, ventricle.

M	C	A	M	T	Y	L	A	H	E
U	A	R	I	C	L	H	Y	L	A
M	I	T	R	A	L	E	C	M	T
U	B	E	T	R	I	I	B	U	R
R	U	R	A	O	R	T	A	R	I
B	H	Y	U	T	H	H	I	M	V
V	E	O	N	I	T	E	R	U	M
H	A	E	T	D	T	A	T	R	I
A	V	E	I	N	R	R	A	M	E
L	E	Y	P	I	A	T	I	E	V

Name ______________________ Date ______________
Course ______________ Instructor ______________

Student Lab Sheet: Assessing the Cardiovascular System

Client's Initials: ______________
Age: ______________
Gender: ______________

Health History

BIOGRAPHICAL DATA:

Current Health Status:
Symptom Analysis (PQRST):

- Chest pain
- Dyspnea
- Cough
- Edema
- Syncope
- Palpitations
- Fatigue
- Extremity changes

Past Health History:

- Childhood illnesses
- Hospitalizations
- Surgeries
- Serious injuries/chronic illness
- Immunizations
- Allergies (food, drugs, environmental)
- Medications
- Recent travel/military service

Family History:

Review of Systems:

- General health status
- HEENT
- Respiratory
- Gastrointestinal
- Genitourinary
- Musculoskeletal
- Neurologic
- Endocrine
- Lymphatic/hematological

Psychosocial Profile:

- Health practices and beliefs/self-care activities
- Typical day
- Nutritional patterns (24-hour recall)
- Activity/exercise patterns
- Recreation, pets, hobbies
- Sleep/rest patterns
- Personal habits (tobacco, alcohol, caffeine, and drugs)
- Occupational health patterns
- Socioeconomic status
- Environmental health patterns
- Roles, relationships, self-concept
- Cultural/religious influences
- Family roles/relationships
- Sexuality patterns
- Social supports
- Stress/coping

Physical Assessment

GENERAL SURVEY:

- Vital signs
- Height
- Weight

Head-to-Toe Scan:

- Integumentary
- HEENT
- Respiratory
- Abdomen
- Genitourinary
- Musculoskeletal
- Neurologic

Assessing the Cardiovascular System

Area/Physical Assessment Skill	Assessment	Normal Findings Developmental/Cultural Variations	Student's Findings
INSPECTION	**Positions: Sitting, supine, left lateral recumbent.**		
Neck vessels: Carotid arteries and jugular veins	Differentiate carotid pulsations from venous pulsations. **Jugular pulsations easily obliterated, affected by position, respirations, undulating wave.** Measure jugular venous pressure with patient at a 45-degree angle at sternal angle (angle of Louis).	Visible carotid pulsation. No neck vein distension. Jugular venous pressure at 45-degree angle < 3 cm. Carotid pulsation with one positive wave. Jugular pulsation undulated.	
Precordium	Note pulsations in apex, LLSB, bases, and xyphoid or epigastric areas.	Positive pulsation noted at apex. Slight pulsation noted at bases in thin adults and children. Slight epigastric pulsations may be noted.	
PALPATION			
Neck vessels: Carotid arteries and jugular veins	**Palpate each carotid separately.** Note rate, rhythm, amplitude, contour, symmetry, elasticity, thrills. **If you feel a carotid thrill, listen for a bruit.** Palpate jugular veins and check direction of fill. Check for abdominojugular (hepatojugular) reflux.	*Carotids:* Rate age dependent; regular rhythm, +2 amplitude, +3 high-output states, equal contour, smooth upstroke with less acute descent; large pulse wave may be seen in elderly and during exercise. Carotids soft and pliable; may be stiff and cordlike in elderly. No thrills. Jugulars easily obliterated and fill appropriately. Negative abdominojugular reflux.	
Precordium	Palpate apex, LLSB, bases, and xyphoid or epigastric areas. Note size, duration, and diffusion of impulses. Note thrills, lifts, or heaves. **If you palpate a thrill, listen for a murmur.**	PMI at apex 1 to 2 cm, nonsustained, or may normally be nonpalpable. Slight epigastric pulsation, no diffusion. No pulsations noted at base and LLSB. Small nonsustained impulses may be palpable at base and LLSB of thin adults and children. PMI may be displaced laterally and to left during last trimester of pregnancy. Increased amplitude in high-output states. No lifts, heaves, or thrills.	

PERCUSSION	**Use indirect (mediate) percussion.**		
Precordium	Percuss from anterior axillary line to sternum at fifth ICS.	Dullness noted th rd, fourth, and fifth ICS to left of sternum at midclavicular line.	
AUSCULTATION	**Listen with bell (light pressure) and diaphragm (heavy pressure) of stethoscope at all sites.**		
Carotids	Listen for bruits with bell of stethoscope. **Have patient hold breath when auscultating for carotid bruits.**	Negative carotid bruits. Carotid bruit may be normal in children and with high-output states.	
Jugular veins	Have patient hold breath when auscultating with bell for venous hums. **To differentiate venous hum from transmitted murmur, remember that venous hum disappears when pressure is applied to jugular vein.**	Negative venous hum. Venous hum may be normal finding in children.	
Precordium	**Auscultate in sitting, supine, and left lateral recumbent positions.**		
Apex: Fifth ICS, left midclavicular line.		*Apex:* Rate/age dependent, rhythm regular, high-pitched, systolic, short duration, 3/6 intensity, $S_1 > S_2$, accentuated S_1 in high-output states.	
LLSB: Fourth to fifth ICS, lateral sternal border	Listen to S_1, S_2, splits, and extra sounds (S_3, S_4, OS ejection click, murmurs, pericardial rubs).	LLSB: S_1 > or = S_2, split S_1 possible.	
Erb's point: third ICS, lateral sternal border	Note rate, rhythm, pitch, intensity, duration, timing in cardiac cycle, quality, location, and radiation.	Base left: $S_1 < S_2$, split S_2 during inspiration. Base right: $S_1 < S_2$.	
Base left: Second ICS, lateral sternal border	**Abnormal aortic murmurs heard best at Erb's point.**	No extra sounds.	
Base right: Second ICS, right sternal border	Grade murmurs on 1 to 6 scale.		
Xyphoid area	**A diastolic murmur or murmur > grade 3/6 is never innocent.**		

(continued)

Assessing the Cardiovascular System (continued)

Pertinent Health History Findings:

Pertinent Physical Assessment Findings:

Nursing Diagnoses (Actual or Potential) With Clustered Data:

Name ______________________	Date ______________
Course ______________________	Instructor ______________

Self-Evaluation Exercise

Cardiovascular System	Yes	No	Needs More Practice
1. Applies knowledge of the cardiovascular system anatomy and physiology in performing a cardiovascular assessment.			
2. Applies growth and development principles as applicable to the cardiovascular system.			
3. Considers cultural variations as indicated when performing a cardiovascular assessment.			
4. Gathers all equipment necessary to perform a cardiovascular assessment.			
5. Obtains history specific to assessment of the cardiovascular system.			
6. Performs a physical assessment of the cardiovascular system, including: • General survey and head-to-toe scan. • Inspection. • Palpation. • Percussion. • Ausculation.			
7. Documents cardiovascular assessment findings.			
8. Identifies normal/abnormal findings.			
9. Clusters pertinent subjective/objective data.			
10. Identifies actual/potential health problems and states them as nursing diagnoses with supporting data.			

Chapter 15

Assessing the Peripheral-Vascular and Lymphatic Systems

Name ________________________ Date ____________

Course ________________ Instructor ________________

1. Anatomy review: Label the following pulse sites.
   - a. Temporal
   - b. Carotid
   - c. Brachial
   - d. Radial
   - e. Ulnar
   - f. Popliteal
   - g. Dorsalis pedis
   - h. Posterior tibial
   - i. Femoral

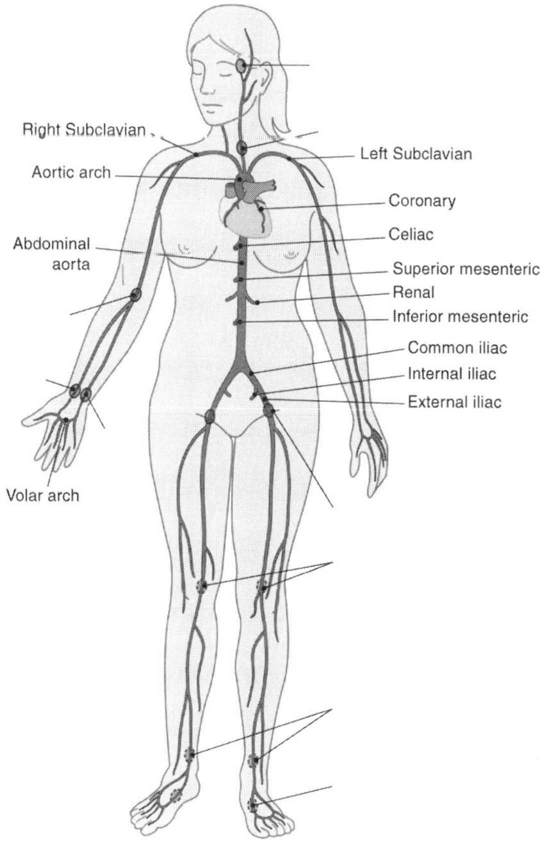

2. Match the structures in the first column to their specific functions in the second column.

Structure	Function
1. Carotid artery	a. Lymphatic tissue found in oropharynx
2. Peyer's patch	b. Drain arms
3. Jugular veins	c. Provides blood supply to brain
4. Thymus	d. Organ in left upper quadrant of abdomen that produces lymphocytes and monocytes
5. Spleen	e. Drain head
6. Subclavian veins	f. Cluster of lymphatic tissue in intestines
7. Femoral artery	g. Drain legs
8. Brachial artery	h. Provides blood supply to legs
9. Tonsils	i. Provides blood supply to arms
10. Iliac veins	j. Lymphatic tissue in thorax that helps with T-cell differentiation

3. You are working in a hypertension (HTN) clinic. Describe the technique you should use to avoid the auscultatory gap when measuring blood pressure (BP).

____

____

4. What three positions should the patient be in when you measure for orthostatic drops in BP?

____

5. If your patient has a true orthostatic drop, what changes would you expect to find?

____

____

6. You are doing a vascular assessment on Joe McCloskey, a 70-year-old man with a history of diabetes mellitus and peripheral-vascular disease. Identify five characteristics you should include in the pulse assessment.

____

____

7. Considering Mr. McCloskey's age, what would you expect to be a normal variation of the pulse assessment associated with aging?

____

8. Mr. McCloskey tells you that he has an ulcer on his foot caused by vascular problems and diabetes. How do the signs of arterial insufficiency differ from those of venous insufficiency?

____

____

9. What additional test could you do to assess the circulation in Mr. McCloskey's feet?

____

10. Patty Hoffman, age 14, has mononucleosis and associated lymphadenopathy. Name five characteristics that you should note when describing palpable lymph nodes.

____

____

11. What would you expect to find when assessing Patty's lymph nodes?

____

____

12. Lymph nodes normally vary depending on the person's age. What variations would you expect to see in a young child? In an older adult?

____

____

13. Although your assessment focuses on the peripheral-vascular and lymphatic systems, all systems are related. What assessment findings (subjective or objective) show the relationship between the peripheral-vascular and lymphatic systems and other systems?

____

____

____

Name ______________________ Date ______________

Course ______________ Instructor ______________

Abnormal Case Study: Morris Hart

Morris Hart, a 58-year-old, married African American man, is admitted to your medical unit. He has a history of coronary artery disease, HTN, and diabetes. Mr. Hart describes himself as being "in fairly good health" and mentions that he has worked hard to develop a healthy lifestyle. He hasn't had any more "chest pain attacks" and he has been monitoring his BP and his blood sugar at home. He is admitted because of intermittent claudication and pain in his left leg and small open ulcers on two of his toes.

Helpful Hint: Claudication alone is thought to be benign in regard to limb loss, and with lifestyle modification, symptoms remain the same or improve in 80 percent of patients.

Health History

CHIEF COMPLAINT:

"My left leg hurts, and I have two sores on my toes that won't heal."

Symptom Analysis:

P—Patient states that pain occurs sooner when he is walking on an incline or climbing stairs. Reports that pain disappears when he stops walking. He hasn't taken any medications to relieve the pain.

Q—Patient describes pain as a "tightening pressure" and says he sometimes has a sharp, "cramp-like" sensation. Says that several months ago pain occurred only occasionally, but now it occurs almost daily and after walking much shorter distances. It is affecting his ability to do his job.

R—Says that pain is in muscles of calves, thighs, and buttocks on both sides, but left side is worse than right. Besides leg pain, patient has noticed a small ulcer on great toe of his left foot.

T—Has had increasing difficulty walking over past 6 months. Pain usually starts after he has walked about 50 yards and lasts 10 minutes after he stops walking.

Current Health Status:

- *Intermittent claudication:* Progressive worsening over last 6 months that is more painful in left leg.
- *HTN:* Patient is on an angiotensin-converting enzyme inhibitor medication to control BP. He takes his BP two to three times weekly using a home monitor kit. His usual reading is about 150 to 160/90 mm Hg.
- *Diabetes mellitus:* Patient has been a diabetic for 10 years. He takes an oral hyperglycemic agent twice daily and monitors his diet to keep blood glucose under control. Reports a usual fasting blood glucose (before breakfast) between 150 and 160 mg/dL.
- *Coronary artery disease:* Patient had a few episodes of chest pain several years ago and was diagnosed with stable angina. Has sublingual nitroglycerin to take if pain occurs and takes one aspirin daily. Hasn't needed nitroglycerin for more than 1 year.
- *Smoking:* Smoked two packs of cigarettes a day for 30 years. After chest pain episodes, he tried several times to stop smoking but has only been able to cut down to one pack a day.

Family History:

- Father died of an acute myocardial infarction at age 57.
- Mother is alive but had a stroke at age 62 and has been a type 2 diabetic for 15 years.

Psychosocial Profile:

- *Nutritional patterns:* Tries hard to follow diet dietitian gave him when he was first diagnosed with diabetes. Says it has been hard to "eat healthy" lately and admits to cheating on his diet lately. Attributes his current high blood glucose values to this situation. Mrs. Hart has been nagging him to watch his diet.

- *Recreation/hobbies:* Is too busy to have any hobbies. After work, he eats dinner and watches TV.
- *Occupational health patterns:* Mr. Hart is a salesman for a drug company, which requires long hours and frequent out-of-town travel.
- *Environmental health patterns:* Lives in a ranch-style house in suburbs. Has central heating and air conditioning.
- *Roles/relationships:* Lives with his wife. They have two sons in college who come home summers and holidays. The Harts enjoy going to the movies and out to dinner with friends. They used to take long walks in nice weather, but Mr. Hart's current leg problems have interfered with this activity.

14. From Mr. Hart's history, identify risk factors for vascular disease.

____

____

Physical Assessment

- *General appearance:* Well nourished, in no acute distress, slightly anxious.
- *Vital signs:* Afebrile; pulse 98 beats per minute (BPM), regular; respirations 16/min, unlabored, BP 150/96 mm Hg; weight 200 lb (overweight); height 5 feet, 9 inches; body mass index (BMI) 29.
- *Inspection:*
  - *Head and neck:* No jugular vein distension.
  - *Upper extremities:* Skin color uniform; capillary refill < 3 seconds; no edema or skin lesions.
  - *Abdomen:* No visible pulsations.
  - *Lower extremities:*
  - Feet pale on elevation and dusky red on dependency, worse in left leg.
  - Skin thin and shiny.
  - Patchy hair loss.
  - No varicosities.
  - No edema.
  - Nails thickened.
  - Ulcer on lateral side of great toe measuring 2 cm x 2 cm.
- *Palpation:*
  - *Head and neck:* Temporal and carotid arteries +2 bilaterally.
  - *Upper extremities:* Brachial, radial, and ulnar pulses easily palpable (+2); no abnormal filling on Allen's test.
  - *Abdomen:* No abdominal pulsatile mass noted.
  - *Lower extremities:*
  - Femoral and popliteal pulses easily palpable (+2) bilaterally.
  - Dorsalis pedis and posterior tibial pulses absent.
  - Feet and legs cool, especially on left side.
  - Calf circumference: left leg = 20 cm; right leg = 20.5 cm.
- *Auscultation:*
  - *Head and neck:* No carotid bruits.
  - *Upper extremities:* BP 156/96 mm Hg right arm; 158/94 mm Hg left arm.
  - *Abdomen:* No vascular sounds auscultated.

15. What findings suggest arterial insufficiency?

____

____

16. What additional assessment test would help evaluate the circulation in Mr. Hart's lower extremities?

____

17. Before treating the lesions on Mr. Hart's toes, it is essential to assess blood flow in the lower extremities. Why?

____

____

18. Cluster the supporting data for the following nursing diagnoses:

a. Pain related to ischemia.

____

b. Altered tissue perfusion related to decreased arterial blood flow.

____

c. Impaired skin integrity related to decreased peripheral perfusion.

____

19. Identify any additional nursing diagnoses for Mr. Hart.

____

____

20. What health promotion topics should you teach Mr. Hart?

____

21. Describe a walking program for Mr. Hart and its role.

____

____

22. Teaching about leg and foot care is an important intervention for patients with peripheral arterial occlusive disease. List key elements of a teaching plan for Mr. Hart.

____

____

23. *Word jumble:* Unscramble the following words. Then unscramble the circled letters to complete the sentence: Arteries are auscultated for ________________.

1. A H I C A (B) L R
2. F O K K O R O F (T)
3. G E R B E (R) U E D S I S A E
4. Y A N R D (U) A S S E D I S A E
5. N A M S O H G N S (I)
6. L E L N A E S T T
7. O P I L E T P L A
8. R F O L A M E
9. I N E V
10. T E R A Y R

Name ______________________________ Date ______________

Course ______________________ Instructor ______________________

Student Lab Sheet: Assessing the Peripheral-Vascular and Lymphatic Systems

Client's Initials: ______________________

Age: ______________________

Gender: ______________________

Health History

BIOGRAPHICAL DATA:

Current Health Status:
Symptom Analysis (PQRST):

- Swelling
- Limb pain
- Changes in sensations
- Fatigue

Past Health History:

- Childhood illnesses
- Hospitalizations
- Surgeries
- Serious injuries/chronic illness
- Immunizations
- Allergies (food, drugs, environmental)
- Medications (prescribed and over-the-counter [OTC])
- Recent travel/military service

Family History:

Review of Systems:

- General health status
- Head, eyes, ears, nose, and throat (HEENT)
- Integumentary
- Respiratory
- Cardiovascular
- Gastrointestinal
- Genitourinary
- Musculoskeletal
- Neurologic
- Endocrine
- Lymphatic/hematological

Psychosocial Profile:

- Health practices and beliefs/self-care activities
- Typical day
- Nutritional patterns (24-hour recall)
- Activity/exercise patterns
- Recreation, pets, hobbies
- Sleep/rest patterns
- Personal habits (tobacco, alcohol, caffeine, and drugs)
- Occupational health patterns
- Socioeconomic status
- Environmental health patterns
- Roles, relationships, self-concept
- Cultural/religious influences
- Family roles/relationships
- Sexuality patterns
- Social supports
- Stress/coping

Physical Assessment

GENERAL SURVEY:

- Vital signs
- Height
- Weight

Head-to-Toe Scan:

- General health status
- Integumentary
- HEENT
- Respiratory
- Abdomen
- Genitourinary
- Neurologic

Assessing the Peripheral-Vascular and Lymphatic Systems

Area/Physical Assessment Skill	Assessment	Normal Findings Developmental/Cultural Variations	Student's Findings
INSPECTION	**Position: Supine and sitting.**		
Upper extremities	Note color, edema, erythema, red streaks, lesions, and capillary refill. **Look for edema on most dependent parts of body.** **If edema present, weigh patient daily. Grade edema grade +1 to +4.**	Skin color uniform; no erythema, red streaks, edema, or lesions.	
Abdomen	Note shape, arterial pulsation, increased venous pattern, ascites. **If ascites present, do fluid wave test or test for shifting dullness.** ***If large, diffuse arterial pulsation present, do not palpate abdomen.***	Abdomen flat or slightly rounded. No increased venous pattern or ascites. Slight arterial pulsation noted in epigastric region at midline.	
Lower extremities	Note color, skin condition, hair distribution, varicosities, edema, erythema, red streaks, and lesions. **If edema present, measure calf circumference.** **If varicosities present, check venous valve competence with Trendelenburg test or manual compression test.**	Leg hair evenly distributed; color uniform; no edema, varicosities, erythema, red streaks, or lesions.	
Pulses: Carotid Temporal Brachial Radial Ulnar Femoral Popliteal Dorsalis pedis Posterior Tibialis Extremities	**Use light palpation with finger pads.** Note rate, rhythm, equality, amplitude, elasticity, and thrills. Grade amplitude: 0 = Absent. 1 = Weak. 3 = Full. 4 = Bounding. **If thrill is present, listen for a bruit.** If indicated, do Allen test to assess arterial flow to hands. If indicated, do color change test or measure ankle-brachial index to assess arterial flow to legs. If thrombus or thrombophlebitis suspected, test Homans' sign.	Pulses rate/age dependent, regular, equal, +2, arteries soft and pliable. No thrills. Negative Homans' sign. **Document pulse amplitudes on a stick figure.**	

	Assess capillary refill and skin temperature.	Positive capillary refill < 3 seconds. Extremities warm bilaterally.	
Lymph nodes: Cervical Axillary Epitrochlear Inguinal (horizontal and vertical) Popliteal	Note size, shape, symmetry, tenderness, mobility, consistency, delineation, location, erythema, warmth, or increased vascularity.	Lymph nodes not palpable. If node is palpable, normal characteristics include: <1 cm; firm; nontender; round or oval; borders well defined; mobile; no erythema, warmth, or increased vascularity.	
AUSCULTATION	**Use bell of stethoscope.**		
Arteries	Auscultate for bruits.	No bruits.	
BP	Measure BP in both arms, supine, sitting, and, standing. **Avoid auscultatory gap by palpating brachial pulse and inflating cuff until pulse is obliterated, then reinflate cuff 30 mm Hg above the point where pulse was obliterated.** Note orthostatic drop of BP **(decrease of systolic by 10 to 15 mm Hg with increase in pulse rate).** Note pulse pressure **(difference between systolic and diastolic).**	Normal BP age dependent. Adult: systolic < 140 mm Hg, diastolic < 90 mm Hg. **Pulse pressure is one-third of systolic pressure.** No orthostatic drop. **If BP heard down to "0," retake BP and listen for Korotkoff sounds 1, 4 (first diastolic), and 5, then record all three.**	

(continued)

Assessing the Peripheral-Vascular and Lymphatic Systems (continued)

Pertinent Health History Findings:

Pertinent Physical Assessment Findings:

Nursing Diagnoses (Actual or Potential) With Clustered Data:

Name ______________________________ Date ______________

Course ______________________ Instructor ______________________

Self-Evaluation Exercise

Peripheral-Vascular and Lymphatic Systems	Yes	No	Need More Practice
1. Applies knowledge of peripheral-vascular and lymphatic systems anatomy and physiology in performing an assessment of the peripheral-vascular and lymphatic systems.			
2. Applies growth and development principles as applicable to the peripheral-vascular and lymphatic systems.			
3. Considers cultural variations as indicated when performing a peripheral-vascular and lymphatic assessment.			
4. Gathers all equipment necessary to perform a peripheral-vascular and lymphatic systems assessment.			
5. Obtains history specific to assessment of the peripheral-vascular and lymphatic systems.			
6. Performs a physical assessment of the peripheral-vascular and lymphatic systems, including: • General survey and head-to-toe scan. • Inspection. • Palpation. • Auscultation.			
7. Documents peripheral-vascular and lymphatic system assessment findings.			
8. Identifies normal/abnormal findings.			
9. Clusters pertinent subjective/objective data.			
10. Identifies actual/potential health problems and states them as nursing diagnoses with supporting data.			

Chapter 16

Assessing the Breasts

Name ______________________ Date __________

Course ______________________ Instructor ______________________

1. Anatomy review: Label the following structures.
   a. Nipple
   b. Tail of Spence
   c. Quadrants
   d. Upper inner
   e. Upper outer
   f. Lower outer
   g. Lower inner
   h. Montgomery's glands
   i. Areola

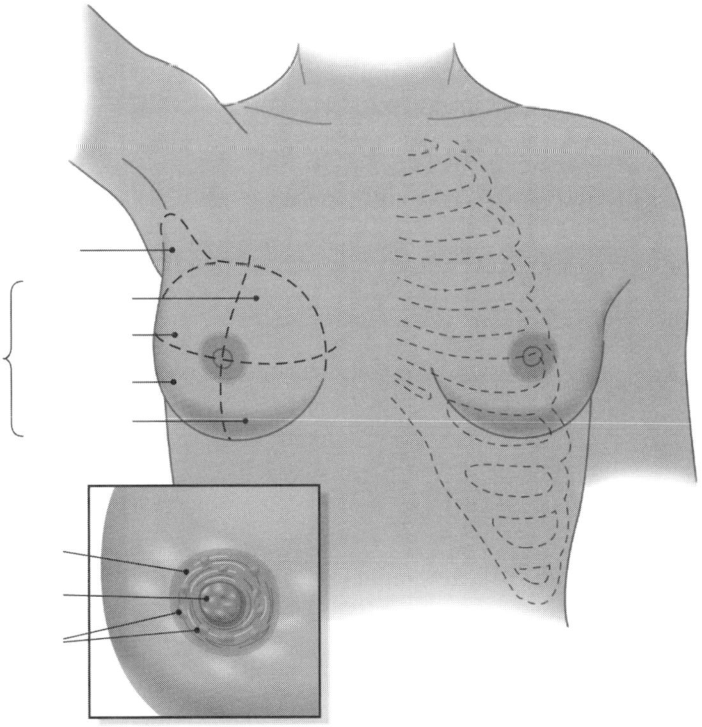

a. Pectoralis major muscle
b. Serratus anterior muscle
c. Adipose tissue
d. Cooper's ligament
e. Lobe
f. Lobule
g. Lactiferous duct

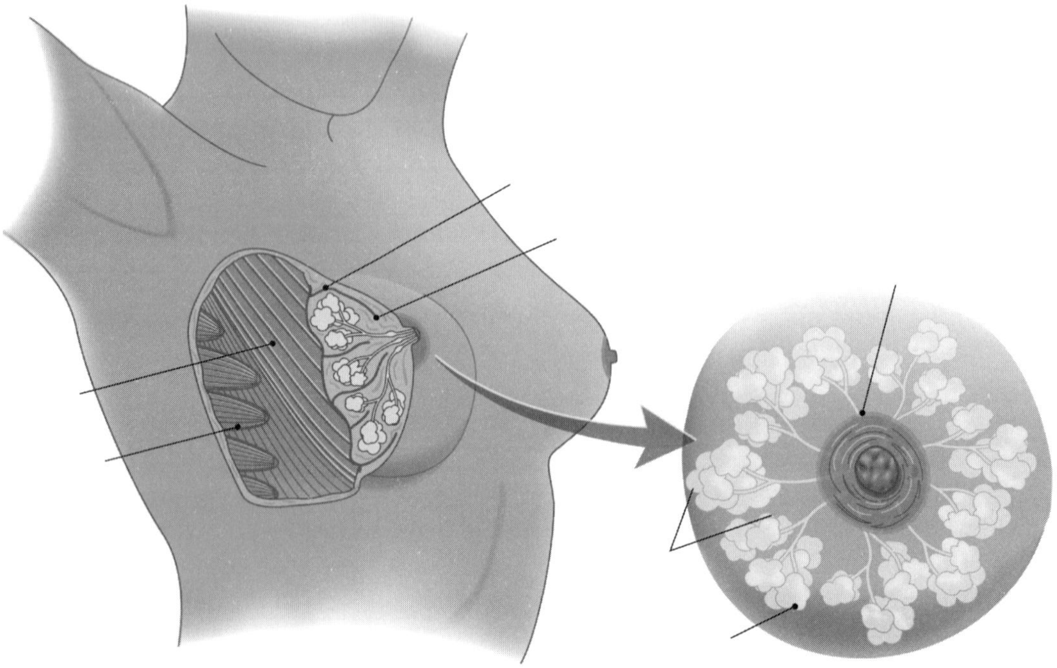

2. Match the structures in the first column to their descriptions in the second column.

Structure	Description
1. Acini	a. Supports breast
2. Lactiferous ducts	b. Sebaceous glands
3. Montgomery's tubercles	c. Produce milk
4. Areola	d. Carry milk from glands
5. Cooper's ligament	e. Dark area surrounding nipple

3. Martha Polanski, age 40, is scheduled for her annual clinical breast exam. List three health history questions that would help you identify her risk factors.

____

____

____

4. You review breast self-exam (BSE) techniques with Mrs. Polanski. When should you advise her to perform BSE?

____

5. You should inspect the breast from several different angles. What four positions should the patient be in during your inspection?

____

____

6. You discover a 1-cm mass in Mrs. Polanski's left breast. What characteristics should you include when describing this mass?

____

____

7. What would you expect to find if the breast mass were malignant?

____

____

8. You should also palpate for lymph node enlargement. Match the lymph nodes in the first column to their appropriate sites in the second column.

Lymph Node	**Site**
1. Central	a. Inner aspect of humerus
2. Anterior	b. Subscapular
3. Lateral	c. High in axilla
4. Posterior	d. Pectoral

9. Although your assessment focuses on the breasts, all systems are related. What assessment findings (subjective or objective) show the relationship between the breasts and other systems?

____

____

____

Name ________________ Date ________________

Course ________________ Instructor ________________

Abnormal Case Study: Mary Jane Marshall

Mary Jane Marshall, 45 years old, is scheduled for a lumpectomy of a possibly malignant breast mass. She is married, has two children ages 14 and 12, and works as a freelance commercial artist. She is accompanied by her husband, who seems supportive and concerned. Mrs. Marshall discovered the breast mass during a BSE 2 weeks ago. She is anxious and on the verge of tears, stating, "I'm so afraid it might be cancer."

Health History

CURRENT HEALTH STATUS:

Breast mass discovered during BSE.

Past Health History:

- No history of breast disease or uterine, ovarian, or colon cancer.
- Menarche age 11.
- Para 2, gravida 2.

Family History:

- Mother and aunt had breast cancer.

Physical Assessment

- Breast mass 4 cm, nontender, irregular, hard, and immobile.
- Anxious, nervous, and tearful.

10. What factors put Mrs. Marshall at risk for breast cancer?

____

____

11. Considering Mrs. Marshall's findings, what additional area should you assess?

____

12. Cluster the supporting data for the following nursing diagnoses:

    a. Risk for pain related to surgical incision.

    ____

    b. Fear related to possible diagnosis of cancer.

    ____

    c. Risk for body image disturbance related to loss of body part.

    ____

13. Identify any additional nursing diagnoses for Mrs. Marshall.

____

____

14. *Word jumble:* Unscramble the following words. Then unscramble the circled letters to complete the sentence: The most frequent site of breast cancer in women is the

_______________.

1. S G T (E) P A
2. T (A) S M (T) S I I
3. (F) A M B E N R (O) O D I A
4. O A (E) A R L
5. (P) N (I) E L P
6. I I N (C) A
7. C O A M Y G (N) T (S) E A I

Name ______________________ Date ______________

Course ______________________ Instructor ______________________

Student Lab Sheet: Assessing the Breasts

Client's Initials: ______________________

Age: ______________________

Gender: ______________________

Health History

BIOGRAPHICAL DATA:

Current Health Status:
Symptom Analysis (PQRST):

- Lump or mass
- Pain or tenderness
- Nipple discharge

Past Health History:

- Childhood illnesses
- Hospitalizations
- Surgeries
- Serious injuries/chronic illness
- Immunizations
- Allergies (food, drugs, environmental)
- Medications (prescribed and over-the-counter [OTC])
- Recent travel/military service

Family History:

Review of Systems:

- General health status
- Head, eyes, ears, nose, and throat (HEENT)
- Respiratory
- Cardiovascular
- Gastrointestinal
- Genitourinary
- Musculoskeletal
- Neurologic
- Endocrine
- Lymphatic/hematological

Psychosocial Profile:

- Health practices and beliefs/self-care activities
- Typical day
- Nutritional patterns (24-hour recall)
- Activity/exercise patterns
- Recreation, pets, hobbies
- Sleep/rest patterns
- Personal habits (tobacco, alcohol, caffeine, and drugs)
- Occupational health patterns
- Socioeconomic status
- Environmental health patterns
- Roles, relationships, self-concept
- Cultural/religious influences
- Family roles/relationships
- Sexuality patterns
- Social supports
- Stress/coping

Physical Assessment

GENERAL SURVEY:

- Vital signs
- Height
- Weight

Head-to-Toe Scan:

- Integumentary
- HEENT
- Respiratory
- Cardiovascular
- Abdomen
- Genitourinary
- Musculoskeletal
- Neurologic

Assessing the Breasts

Area/Physical Assessment Skill	Assessment	Normal Findings Developmental/Cultural Variations	Student's Findings
INSPECTION	**Positions: Sitting with arms at side, arms over head, hands on hips, or leaning forward, or supine with pillow under shoulder of breast being examined.**		
Breasts	Assess size, shape, symmetry, color. Note visible masses, lesions, edema, and venous pattern. **Have patient press hands together or press hands on hips to check for dimpling or retraction.** Note dominant side.	Breasts lobular, symmetrical, color consistent with body color. No masses, lesions, edema, dimpling, retraction, or orange-peel skin. May normally be slightly asymmetrical. Adolescent girls may have asymmetrical breasts as they go through puberty. Adolescent boys may have gynecomastia. During pregnancy, breasts enlarge, venous pattern increases, and areola and nipple darken in color. Postmenopausal breasts lose elasticity and are more pendulous.	
Nipple and areola	Note color, shape, symmetry, inversion/eversion, discharge, masses, lesions, and direction of nipples. Inspect for supernumerary nipples.	Nipples and areola symmetrical, round, and darker than breast tissue. Color lighter in fair-skinned and darker in dark-skinned women. No masses, lesions, or discharge. Spontaneous discharge normal during pregnancy and lactation. Symmetrical nipple direction, usually lateral and upward. Nipples may be everted, flat, or inverted, but should be symmetrical. No supernumerary nipples.	
Axilla	Note color, lesions, masses, and hair distribution.	Skin intact, no lesions or rashes. Hair growth appropriate for patient's age and sex.	
PALPATION	**Use finger pads of three middle fingers, making small circles with light, medium, and deep pressure.**		
Breasts	**Palpate from clavicle to sixth to seventh intercostal space (ICS) and from sternum to midaxillary line. Use vertical strip, pie wedge, or circular method.**	Breast consistency depends on a woman's developmental stage.	

	Note texture, consistency, tenderness, or masses.	Premenopausal breast more firm and elastic; breasts during pregnancy and lactation firm and tender; postmenopausal breasts less firm and elastic with stringy ducts. Nontender, but may be tender and nodular premenstrually.	
Nipple and areola	Note elasticity, discharge, or tenderness. ***Unless pregnant or lactating, spontaneous discharge is abnormal and warrants follow-up.***	No masses or lesions. Nipple elastic, nontender, no discharge or white sebaceous secretion with nipple compression. Pregnant or lactating women may have milky discharge.	
Axilla and clavicular nodes: Central Anterior Posterior Lateral Epitrochlear Supraclavicular Infraclavicular	Note palpable nodes, location, tenderness, size, shape, consistency, mobility, borders, and temperature.	Lymph nodes nonpalpable, nontender.	

(continued)

Assessing the Breasts (continued)

Pertinent Health History Findings:

Pertinent Physical Assessment Findings:

Nursing Diagnoses (Actual or Potential) With Clustered Data:

Name ______________________ Date ____________

Course ______________ Instructor ______________

Self-Evaluation Exercise

Breast Assessment	Yes	No	Needs More Practice
1. Applies knowledge of anatomy and physiology of the breast in performing an assessment of the breast.			
2. Applies growth and development principles as applicable to the breast.			
3. Considers cultural variations as indicated when performing a breast assessment.			
4. Gathers all equipment necessary to perform a breast assessment.			
5. Obtains history specific to assessment of the breast.			
6. Performs a physical assessment of the breast, including: • General survey and head-to-toe scan. • Inspection. • Palpation.			
7. Documents breast assessment findings.			
8. Identifies normal/abnormal findings.			
9. Clusters pertinent subjective/objective data.			
10. Identifies actual/potential health problems and states them as nursing diagnoses with supporting data.			

Chapter 17

Assessing the Abdomen

Name ______________________ Date __________

Course ______________ Instructor ______________

1. Anatomy review: Label the following structures.
   a. Liver
   b. Gallbladder
   c. Small intestine
   d. Ascending colon
   e. Transverse colon
   f. Descending colon
   g. Stomach
   h. Appendix
   i. Urinary bladder
   j. Spleen

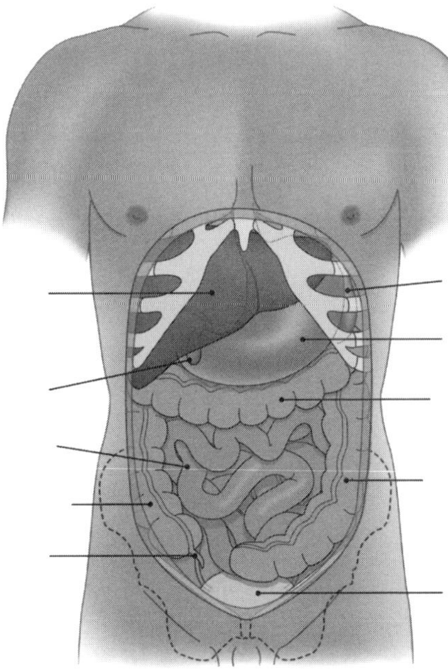

2. Match the structures in the first column to their descriptions in the second column.

Structure	Description
1. Esophagus	a. Primary site for digestion
2. Pancreas	b. Muscular tube that connects mouth to stomach
3. Small intestines	c. Stores bile
4. Gallbladder	d. Secretes insulin, glucagons, and digestive enzymes
5. Appendix	e. Connects small and large intestines
6. Ileocecal valve	f. Common site of infection
7. Liver	g. Reabsorbs water
8. Large intestines	h. Produce saliva and amylase
9. Stomach	i. Churns food and secretes intrinsic factor and hydrochloric acid
10. Salivary glands	j. Primary function is metabolism and detoxification

3. Place the following structures in the correct quadrants.

- Liver ______
- Gallbladder ______
- Pancreas ______
- Stomach ______
- Spleen ______
- Cecum ______
- Appendix ______
- Sigmoid colon ______
- Transverse colon ______
- Ascending colon ______
- Descending colon ______

4. Match the origin of pain in the first column to the referred area of pain in the second column.

Origin of Pain	Referred Area of Pain
1. Ruptured spleen	a. Scapula
2. Cholecystitis	b. Flank and thighs
3. Abdominal aortic aneurysm	c. Shoulder
4. Early appendicitis	d. Low back
5. Renal problems	e. Umbilical area

5. Lou Walker, age 63, had a colon resection 3 days ago. He is NPO and has a nasogastric tube connected to low suction. You begin his abdominal assessment with inspection. What three movements should you look for when inspecting the abdomen?

______

6. After inspecting Mr. Walker's abdomen, you auscultate it. What is the rationale for performing auscultation before palpating the abdomen?

7. You have trouble auscultating Mr. Walker's bowel sounds. How long should you auscultate before charting that bowel sounds are absent?

8. Before charting that Mr. Walker has absent bowel sounds, listen over the ileocecal valve. Where is this site located, and what is the rationale for listening over it?

9. Mr. Walker's abdomen is distended, and his bowel sounds are hypoactive. How do you explain these findings?

10. Name two causes for hypoactive or absent bowel sounds.

11. Name two causes of hyperactive bowel sounds.

12. Bill Dwyer, age 56, has been diagnosed with early cirrhosis. Abdominal assessment includes percussion of the liver for size. What test would help you locate the lower border of the liver?

13. What percussion sound would you expect to elicit over the liver?

14. Mr. Dwyer's liver measures 14 cm at the midclavicular line. What is the normal liver size at the midclavicular line?

15. Brian Duffy, a 20-year-old college student, comes to the ED after being injured during a lacrosse game. He presents with left upper quadrant pain. You assess for splenic enlargement and find that his spleen is palpable in the left upper quadrant at the costal margin. Is this a normal finding? Why or why not?

16. You assess Brian's spleen further through percussion. Where do you percuss to locate the spleen?

17. Although your assessment focuses on the abdomen, all systems are related. What assessment findings (subjective or objective) show the relationship between the abdomen and other systems?

____

____

____

Name ______________________ Date ____________

Course ____________________ Instructor ____________________

Abnormal Case Study: Larry Petroski

Larry Petroski, age 25, is admitted to the ED with complaints of nausea, vomiting, and abdominal pain. He is bent over and walking slowly. He states, "I think I have food poisoning." Because his problem is acute, you perform a focused health history.

Health History

CHIEF COMPLAINT:

"I think I have food poisoning."

Symptom Analysis:

P—Standing up makes pain worse, and nothing makes it better.

Q—Describes pain as "sharp and constant."

R—Patient states, "I'm having such pain in my belly." Says that pain was initially around umbilical area, then shifted to right lower quadrant. Denies any radiation.

S—States pain is 10 on the 0-to-10 scale.

T—States that pain started acutely around 10 A.M. and has progressively worsened. He was brought to ED at 1 P.M.

Current Health History:

Patient states, "I am always healthy and never had any problems with my belly before."

Past Health History:

- This is patient's first hospital admission.
- No previous health problems.
- Takes no medications.

Family History:

- Mother died of lung cancer.
- Father alive and well with no health problems.
- No siblings.

Psychosocial Profile:

- *Nutritional patterns:* States that he was able to eat his usual breakfast (cereal and milk) at 8 A.M. Abdominal pain started at 10 A.M., then nausea and vomiting at 10:30 A.M. States that he thinks he has food poisoning.
- *Recreation/hobbies:* Enjoys riding his snowmobile and motorcycle and taking long walks along beach with his wife.
- *Occupational health patterns:* Works as an auto mechanic.
- *Environmental health patterns:* Lives in a suburban city in a one-story house near the ocean.
- *Roles/relationships:* Lives with his wife and daughter and spends a great deal of time with daughter. Is active in local church.

Helpful Hint: In gastroenteritis, nausea and vomiting occur before onset of abdominal pain; in appendicitis, the opposite occurs.

Physical Assessment

- *General appearance:* Appears in obvious distress with his body bent over and his arms covering his abdomen.
- *Vital signs:* Temperature 37.9°C; pulse 89 beats per minute (BPM); respirations 24/min; blood pressure (BP) 139/70 mm Hg.
- *Mental status:* Alert and oriented x 4.
- *Urine:* Yellow and without sediment.
- *Leg edema:* No edema present throughout the body.
- *Inspection:*
  - Abdomen uniformly tan in color.
  - No striae, bruises, or hernias noted; umbilicus centered.
  - Abdomen flat and symmetrical without distension.
  - No aortic pulsations; peristalsis noted.
  - Abdominal respiratory pattern shallow with increased respiratory rate.

- *Auscultation:*
  - Hypoactive bowel sounds in all four quadrants.
  - No bruits, friction rubs, or venous hums.
- *Percussion:*
  - Liver span 7.0 cm right midclavicular line.
  - Unable to percuss bladder or spleen.
  - Negative costovertebral angle tenderness.
- *Palpation:*
  - Light and deep palpation could not be performed on Mr. Petroski because of abdominal pain. Consequently, many of the palpation tests were limited to the essential test, which included the following results:
  - Muscle guarding in the right lower quadrant.
  - Tenderness in the right lower quadrant.

ADDITIONAL ASSESSMENT DATA:

- Rebound tenderness at McBurney's point.
- Positive iliopsoas muscle test.
- Positive obturator muscle test.
- Positive cutaneous hypersensitivity in right lower quadrant.
- Positive Rovsing's sign.

18. Because Mr. Petroski has an abdominal problem, how would you explain the shallow respiratory pattern and increase in respiratory rate?

____

____

19. Mr. Petroski ate breakfast at 8 A.M. What is the importance of identifying the time he last ate?

____

____

20. What additional question should you ask Mr. Petroski if he is scheduled for surgery or will be receiving any medication?

____

____

21. Which of Mr. Petroski's vital signs are abnormal, and what are the causes of these variations?

____

____

22. What physical findings indicate appendicitis?

____

____

____

23. Mr. Petroski was diagnosed as having appendicitis, and he was scheduled for emergency surgery. Cluster the supporting data for the following nursing diagnoses for him:

    a. Pain: Acute related to obstruction of the appendix with inflammation.

    ____

    b. Alteration in comfort: Nausea and vomiting related to stimulation of vomiting center from pain.

    ____

    c. Potential for fluid volume defect related to nausea and vomiting.

    ____

24. Your first priority nursing diagnosis is Pain: Acute related to obstruction of the appendix with inflammation. Select some appropriate preoperative nursing actions.

    ____

    ____

25. One complication of appendicitis is peritonitis. What data should you obtain to ascertain if Mr. Petroski's appendix has ruptured?

    ____

    ____

26. Identify any additional nursing diagnoses for this patient.

    ____

    ____

27. *Word jumble:* Unscramble the following words. Then unscramble the circled letter to complete the sentence: The area of tenderness in acute appendicitis is ____________.

    1. (R) L V I E
    2. S (P) T L A S I E R I S
    3. E R A (T) (S) I
    4. L E A (M) E N
    5. (U) F L S A T
    6. Y H (C) E M
    7. R O G (B) (Y) I M R O B
    8. S I C T E A S
    9. H A (E) R I D A R
    10. T M I (O) C A S A T (N)
    11. E (N) L P S E
    12. H S I C R O R (I) S

Name ______________________________ Date ______________

Course ______________________ Instructor ______________________

Student Lab Sheet: Assessing the Abdomen

Client's Initials: ______________________

Age: ______________________

Gender: ______________________

Health History

BIOGRAPHICAL DATA:

Current Health Status:
Symptom Analysis (PQRST):

- Elimination pattern: Frequency, color, and consistency of stool
- Abdominal pain
- Nausea and vomiting
- Weight changes
- Appetite changes

Past Health History:

- Childhood illnesses
- Hospitalizations
- Surgeries
- Serious injuries/chronic illness
- Immunizations
- Allergies (food, drugs, environmental)
- Medications (prescribed and over-the-counter [OTC])
- Recent travel/military service

Family History:

Review of Systems:

- General health status
- Head, eyes, ears, nose, and throat (HEENT)
- Respiratory
- Cardiovascular
- Genitourinary
- Musculoskeletal
- Neurologic
- Endocrine
- Lymphatic/hematological

Psychosocial Profile:

- Health practices and beliefs/self-care activities
- Typical day
- Nutritional patterns (24-hour recall)
- Activity/exercise patterns
- Recreation, pets, hobbies
- Sleep/rest patterns
- Personal habits (tobacco, alcohol, caffeine, and drugs)
- Occupational health patterns
- Socioeconomic status
- Environmental health patterns
- Roles, relationships, self-concept
- Cultural/religious influences
- Family roles/relationships
- Sexuality patterns
- Social supports
- Stress/coping

Physical Assessment

GENERAL SURVEY:

- Vital signs
- Height
- Weight

Head-to-Toe Scan:

- General health status
- Integumentary
- HEENT
- Respiratory
- Cardiovascular
- Genitourinary
- Musculoskeletal
- Neurologic

Assessing the Abdomen

Area/Physical Assessment Skill	Assessment	Normal Findings Developmental/Cultural Variations	Student's Findings
INSPECTION	**Have patient void before exam.** **Inspect from side and foot of bed.** **Position: Supine.**		
Abdomen	Note size, shape, and symmetry of abdomen. Note condition of skin, color, lesions, scars, striae, superficial veins, and hair distribution. Note abdominal movements: respiratory, pulsation, and peristalsis. Note position, contour, color, and herniation of umbilicus. Have patient raise head off bed, then check for bulges (hernias).	Skin color consistent or slightly lighter than exposed areas. No lesions, striae, superficial veins, scars, rashes, or discoloration. Hair distribution appropriate for patient's age and gender. Abdomen flat or slightly rounded and symmetrical, no bulges or hernias. Positive respiratory movements, slight pulsation noted in epigastric region, no peristaltic waves. Umbilicus midline, inverted, no discoloration or discharge. Pregnant patient may have increased pigmentation at midline (linea nigra), striae, diastasis recti, and upward and outward displacement of umbilicus. Children also may have diastasis recti.	
AUSCULTATION	**Always auscultate before palpating. Palpation may alter bowel sounds.** **Use diaphragm of stethoscope for bowel sounds and friction rubs.** **Use bell for vascular sounds.**		
Abdomen Liver Arteries	Listen for bowel sounds in each quadrant. Listen for at least 5 minutes before saying bowel sounds are absent. **If having difficulty hearing bowel sounds, listen over ileocecal valve to right of umbilicus in right lower quadrant.**	Soft, medium-pitched bowel sounds every 5 to 15 seconds in all four quadrants. No borborygmi, bruits, hums, or rubs. Lower edge of liver located at costal margin by scratch test.	

	Use scratch test to locate inferior edge of liver. Auscultate for bruits over aorta, renal, iliac, and femoral arteries. If indicated, auscultate for venous hum over liver. If indicated, auscultate for friction rubs over organs.		
PERCUSSION	**Use indirect (mediate) percussion in all four quadrants.**		
Abdominal organs (liver, gallbladder, spleen, kidneys, bladder)	Note areas of tympany, dullness, or tenderness Measure liver size at the right midclavicular line. If enlarged, measure at midsternal line. Locate gastric bubble over stomach. Locate splenic dullness at left midaxillary line. Percuss for bladder dullness at the midline above the symphysis pubis.	Tympany in all four quadrants, dullness over organs. Liver 6 to 12 cm at right midclavicular line; 4 to 8 cm at the midsternal line. Splenic dullness 9th, 10th, 11th ribs at right midaxillary line, < 7 cm. Organs nontender. Dullness in suprapubic area: Full bladder (for other causes, see section on abdominal contour and distension).	
Costovertebral Angle (CVA)	Place nondominant hand over organ. Make a fist with dominant hand. Note any tenderness. Kidney tenderness is assessed at the CVA. If ascites, percuss for shifting dullness. If indicated, use fist (blunt) percussion to assess for organ (liver or gallbladder) tenderness. Check for kidney tenderness at posterior CVA. **Percuss tender areas last.**	Negative CVA tenderness.	
PALPATION	**Begin with light palpation, then do deep, bimanual palpation in all four quadrants.** **If patient tenses (voluntary guarding), have him or her slightly flex knees, or let patient hold your hand as you palpate.**		

(continued)

Assessing the Abdomen (continued)

Area/Physical Assessment Skill	Assessment	Normal Findings Developmental/Cultural Variations	Student's Findings
Aorta	Note size and pulsation.	Aorta 2.5 cm. Slight pulsation palpable. No diffusion.	
Abdominal organs	Use light palpation to identify surface characteristics, tenderness, muscular resistance, and turgor and to put patient at ease. Assess umbilicus for bulges or nodules. ***Do not palpate abdomen if patient has Wilms' tumor, large diffuse pulsations, or history of organ transplant.*** Use deep palpation with bimanual technique to palpate organs (liver, spleen, kidneys, bladder) and masses. Note tenderness, consistency, pulsations, and enlarged organs. Palpate aorta, noting pulsation, size, and diffusion. If indicated, assess for rebound tenderness at McBurney's point, the iliopsoas test, and the obturator test. If fluid, test for fluid wave test. Use ballottement to assess fetal position or masses. Test abdominal reflexes by lightly stroking each quadrant toward the umbilicus. If possible gallbladder disease, assess Murphy's sign. If possible splenic injury or rupture, assess Kehr's and Ballance's signs.	Abdomen soft, nontender, no masses, positive skin turgor, and negative umbilical bulges. Liver nonpalpable or liver's edge palpable at costal margin, firm, smooth, and nontender. Spleen nontender, nonpalpable. Negative rebound. Kidneys usually nonpalpable. Right kidney may be palpable in thin woman. Full bladder may be palpable above the symphsis pubis. Positive slight aortic pulsation, no diffusion, aorta 2.5 cm. Positive abdominal reflexes.	
Inguinal lymph nodes	Use light palpation; palpate horizontal and vertical inguinal nodes. Note size, shape, consistency, tenderness, and mobility.	Inguinal nodes nonpalpable, nontender.	

Pertinent Health History Findings:

Pertinent Physical Assessment Findings:

Nursing Diagnoses (Actual or Potential) With Clustered Data:

Name		Date	
Course		Instructor	

Self-Evaluation Exercise

Abdominal Assessment	Yes	No	Needs More Practice
1. Applies knowledge of anatomy and physiology of the abdomen in performing an assessment of the abdomen.			
2. Applies growth and development principles as applicable to the abdomen.			
3. Considers cultural variations as indicated when performing an abdominal assessment.			
4. Gathers all equipment necessary to perform an abdominal assessment.			
5. Obtains history specific to assessment of the abdomen.			
6. Perform a physical assessment of the abdomen, including: • General survey and head-to-toe scan. • Inspection. • Ausculation. • Percussion. • Palpation.			
7. Documents abdominal assessment findings.			
8. Identifies normal/abnormal findings.			
9. Clusters pertinent subjective/objective data.			
10. Identifies actual/potential health problems and states them as nursing diagnoses with supporting data.			

Chapter 18

Assessing the Female Genitourinary System

Name ______________________________ Date ______________

Course ______________________ Instructor ______________________

1. Anatomy review: Label the following structures.

   a. Prepuce of clitoris
   b. Clitoris
   c. Skene's ducts
   d. Vaginal orifice
   e. Urethral orifice
   f. Labia minora
   g. Labia majora
   h. Bartholin's glands
   i. Perineum
   j. Anus
   k. Hymen

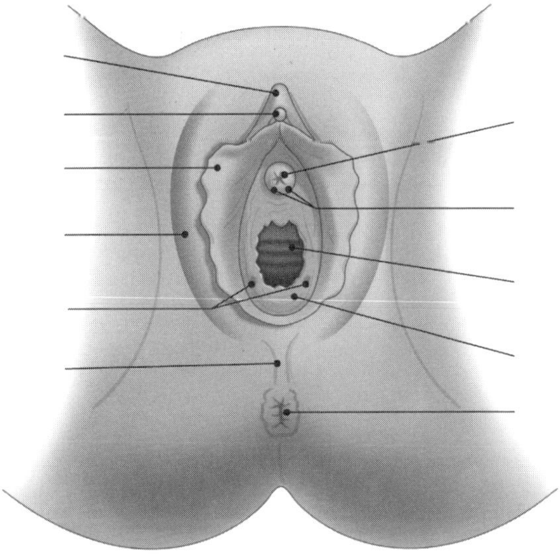

a. Mucous membrane
b. Internal sphincter
c. Uterus
d. Rectum
e. Ovary
f. Posterior fornix of vagina
g. Fallopian tube
h. Cervix
i. Vagina
j. Bladder
k. Anal valves
l. External sphincter
m. Rectal columns
n. Anterior fornix of vagina
o. Symphysis pubis
p. Anus
q. Urethra
r. Sigmoid colon
s. Clitoris
t. Labia minora
u. Labia majora
v. Rectum
w. Peritoneal cavity

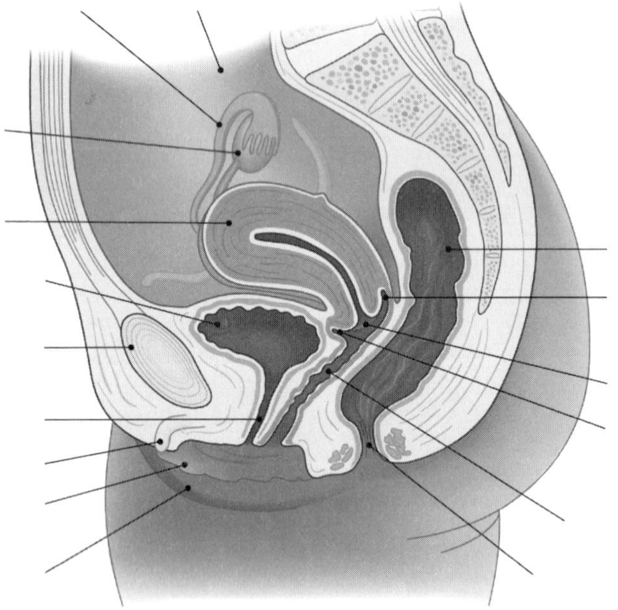

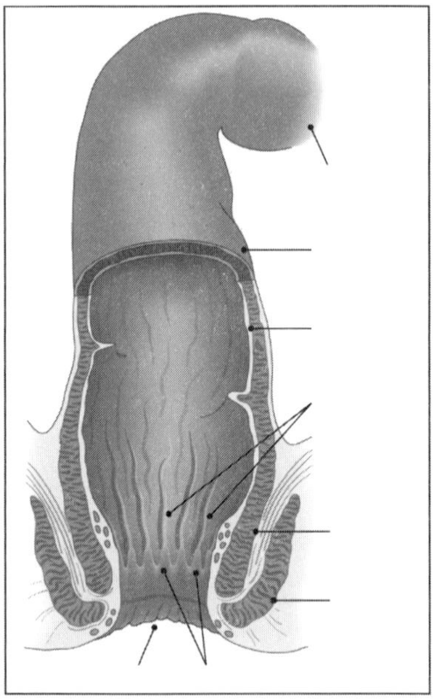

2. Match the structures in the first column to their descriptions in the second column.

Structure	Description
1. Ovaries	a. Muscular sac that stores urine
2. Uterus	b. Muscle layer of uterus
3. Bartholin's gland	c. Ducts from kidneys to bladder
4. Skene's gland	d. Uterine neck that joins to cervix
5. Endometrium	e. Duct from bladder that allows for urine excretion
6. Isthmus	f. Pear-shaped muscular structure for implantation of fertilized ovum
7. Cervix	g. Secrete estrogen, progesterone, and ova
8. Vagina	h. Secretes alkaline mucus that improves viability and motility of sperm

9. Ureters	i. Paraurethral gland that provides lubrication to protect skin
10. Urethra	j. Inner lining of uterus
11. Myometrium	k. Uterine part that extends into vagina
12. Bladder	l. Muscular passageway from cervix to vulva for copulation and menses; also called birth canal

3. Donna Goldstein, age 48, is scheduled for a routine gynecological exam. Mrs. Goldstein states, "I think I'm going through menopause." Name three signs or symptoms that suggest menopause.

____

____

4. Mrs. Goldstein's daughter Michelle, age 18, is also scheduled for an exam. Michelle has never had a gynecological exam. At what age should a woman begin having a routine gynecological exam?

____

5. Michelle asks, "What is a Pap test?"

____

6. Before beginning the exam, what five questions should you ask Michelle?

____

____

____

____

____

7. At what age should an adolescent be referred if she has not reached menarche?

____

8. Because this is Michelle's first gynecological exam, you need to explain what you are doing and why you are doing it. What is the purpose of the internal gynecological exam?

____

____

9. Mrs. Goldstein is parous and Michelle is nulliparous. How would you expect each of their cervices to look?

____

____

10. Match the abnormalities in the first column with their descriptions in the second column.

Abnormality	**Description**
1. Condyloma acuminatum	a. Painful menses
2. Pediculosis pubis	b. Genital warts
3. Trichomonas	c. Painful vesicular lesions
4. Dysmenorrhea	d. Painful intercourse
5. Gonorrhea	e. Greenish gray, watery, frothy, malodorous discharge
6. Amenorrhea	f. Nits
7. Candidiasis	g. Heavy menstrual bleeding
8. Chancre	h. Purulent greenish-yellow discharge
9. Chancroid	i. Grayish-white discharge
10. Menorrhagia	j. Absent menses
11. Genital herpes	k. Cheeselike discharge
12. Dyspareunia	l. Nonpainful, nonscarring syphilitic lesions
13. Chlamydia	m. Painful, scarring pustules or ulcers with yellow discharge

11. Although your assessment focuses on the female genitourinary system, all systems are related. What assessment findings (subjective or objective) show the relationship between the female genitourinary system and other systems?

____

____

____

Name ______________________ Date ______________

Course ______________________ Instructor ______________________

Abnormal Case Study: Helen McCloskey

Helen McCloskey is a 60-year-old, white, single woman with a diagnosis of ovarian mass, possible ovarian cancer. She is scheduled for a total abdominal hysterectomy. As you prepare her for surgery, you observe that she seems anxious. She states, "I'm scared about what the doctor is going to find." She complains of indigestion, nausea, and loss of appetite for the past month.

Health History

CHIEF COMPLAINT:

"For the past month, I've had indigestion and felt sick to my stomach. I don't have any appetite, either."

Symptom Analysis:

P—No identifiable precipitating factor; some relief of indigestion with antacids.

Q—Feels like "constant upset stomach."

R—Located in stomach and lower abdomen; other symptoms are constipation, weight loss, but clothes feel tight.

S—Has become progressively worse, now almost constant.

T—"Started a month ago, but I thought I had a gastrointestinal bug."

Biographical Data:

- Works as a lawyer.
- Health insurance: Blue Cross/Blue Shield.

Current Health Status:

- Denies any major medical problems.
- No prescription medications, using antacids for indigestion, occasional use of aspirin for headache.
- Allergies: No known drug allergies.

Past Health History:

- No surgeries or hospitalizations.
- Menarche at age 11, nulliparous, menopause at age 50.
- Currently not sexually active.
- Last gynecological exam 5 years ago.

Family History:

- Mother died of ovarian cancer at age 70.
- Aunt died of ovarian cancer at age 72.
- Family history of hypertension (HTN) and stroke.

Psychosocial Profile:

- *Nutritional patterns:* Eats on the run, hard to cook for one, diet tends to be high in fat.
- *Personal habits:* No smoking or use of drugs. Occasional use of alcohol (two drinks per month).
- *Environmental health patterns:* Lives alone in single, two-story home in suburbs.
- *Social supports:* Sister lives 20 minutes away and will help after surgery.

12. What presenting symptoms of Ms. McCloskey's are associated with ovarian cancer?

____

____

13. Considering Ms. McCloskey's history, identify any risk factors for ovarian cancer.

____

____

Physical Assessment

- *General appearance:* Appears younger than age 60; affect anxious; communicative and willing to undergo examination.
- *Vital signs:* Temperature 98.8°F; pulse 98 beats per minute (BPM), regular; respirations 22/min, shallow; blood pressure (BP) 160/90 mm Hg; height 5 feet, 4 inches; weight 160 lb.

PELVIC EXAM

- *Skin:* Hair gray and sparse, distribution appropriate for maturation level.
- *Genitalia:*
  - No lesions, other signs of infection, or obvious congenital abnormalities.
  - Cervix clear, pale pink, without lesions, midline; os is patent.
  - No swelling or induration of labia, urethral meatus, Skene's glands, or Bartholin's gland.
  - Vaginal muscle tone strong.
  - Cervix mobile and nontender.
  - Uterus is small, pear-shaped, firm, mobile, nontender, and anteverted.
  - Adnexa: Left ovary nonpalpable, right ovary palpable, enlarged, hard, irregular, and nontender.
- *Abdomen:*
  - Round, positive ascites, decreased bowel sounds, soft and nontender except right lower quadrant.
  - Palpable immobile mass about 8 cm, hard, irregular, and nontender.

14. Considering that Ms. McCloskey has ascites, what other area warrants assessment?

____

____

15. Cluster the supporting data for the following nursing diagnoses:

a. Pain (abdominal discomfort) related to enlarging tumor on ovary.

____

b. Constipation.

____

c. Anxiety related to threat of possible malignancy.

____

16. The following diagnoses are not actual problems and have no supporting data. State the rationale for each potential problem.

    a. Risk for infection related to surgery.

    ____

    b. Risk for ineffective breathing problems related to ascites and surgery.

    ____

    ____

17. Identify any additional nursing diagnoses for Ms. McCloskey.

    ____

    ____

    ____

18. *Word search:* Find the following words in the puzzle: bladder, cervix, gravida, menarche, menses, ovary, parity, puberty, ureter, urethra, vagina.

B	C	P	A	Y	M	P	U	M	L
L	E	V	R	A	E	U	R	E	P
A	R	A	R	N	N	B	E	N	A
D	V	X	E	I	S	L	T	A	R
O	I	A	C	G	E	A	H	R	I
D	X	G	R	A	S	D	R	C	T
E	G	R	A	V	I	D	A	H	Y
R	T	U	R	E	T	E	R	E	G
R	A	P	U	B	E	R	T	Y	H
C	L	A	P	R	M	E	N	S	L

Name ______________________ Date ______________

Course ______________________ Instructor ______________________

Student Lab Sheet: Assessing the Female Genitourinary System

Client's Initials: ______________________

Age: ______________________

Gender: ______________________

Health History

BIOGRAPHICAL DATA:

Current Health Status:
Symptom Analysis (PQRST):

- Vaginal discharge
- Pain
- Lumps/masses
- Dysmenorrhea
- Amenorrhea
- Urinary symptoms

Past Health History:

- Childhood illnesses
- Hospitalizations
- Surgeries
- Serious injuries/chronic illness
- Immunizations
- Allergies (food, drugs, environmental)
- Medications (prescribed and over-the-counter [OTC])
- Recent travel/military service

Family History:

Review of Systems:

- General health status
- Head, eyes, ears, nose, and throat (HEENT)
- Respiratory
- Cardiovascular
- Gastrointestinal
- Musculoskeletal
- Neurologic
- Endocrine
- Lymphatic/hematological

Psychosocial Profile:

- Health practices and beliefs/self-care activities
- Typical day
- Nutritional patterns (24-hour recall)
- Activity/exercise patterns
- Recreation, pets, hobbies
- Sleep/rest patterns
- Personal habits (tobacco, alcohol, caffeine, and drugs)
- Occupational health patterns
- Socioeconomic status
- Environmental health patterns
- Roles, relationships, self-concept
- Cultural/religious influences
- Family roles/relationships
- Sexuality patterns
- Social supports
- Stress/coping

Physical Assessment

GENERAL SURVEY:

- Vital signs
- Height
- Weight

Head-to-Toe Scan:

- General health status
- Integumentary
- HEENT
- Respiratory
- Cardiovascular
- Abdominal
- Musculoskeletal
- Neurologic

Assessing the Female Genitourinary System

Area/Physical Assessment Skill	Assessment	Normal Findings Developmental/Cultural Variations	Student's Findings
INSPECTION	**Position: Lithotomy. Maintain standard precautions, wear gloves.**		
External genitalia	**Have patient void before exam.**		
Labia majora Labia minora Clitoris Urethra Vaginal orifice Skene's glands	Note color, hair distribution, condition of skin, swelling, lesions, polyps, discharge, odor, prolapse, or pubic pediculosis. No lesions, edema, discharge, odor, or prolapse (bladder, uterus, or rectum).	External genitalia intact, pink, and moist; color depends on patient's pigmentation. Hair distribution depends on age and development of patient.	
Bartholin's glands Perineum	Normal cervical discharge depends on menstrual cycle: clear and stretchy before ovulation, white and opaque after ovulation, bloody during menstruation.		
Rectal area	Note condition of skin, inflammation, rashes, excoriation, rectal prolapse, external hemorrhoids, polyps, lesions, fissures, bleeding, and discharge.	Rectal area intact, no inflammation, lesions, prolapse, hemorrhoids, discharge, or bleeding.	
PELVIC EXAM WITH SPECULUM Cervix Vaginal walls	Use warm speculum. Note color, lesions, discharge, bleeding, position, size, shape and symmetry, shape and patency of os. Obtain specimens as indicated. Inspect vaginal walls while withdrawing speculum.	Cervix round, midline, pink, no lesions or discharge, os is slit in parous female, round and closed in nulliparous female. Bluish color seen with pregnancy, paler color seen in postmenopausal women. Vaginal walls pink with rugae, no lesions.	

PALPATION	**Lubricate index and middle fingers of gloved hand. Perform vaginal exam first, then speculum exam, bimanual exam, and rectovaginal exam.**		
Skene's glands, Bartholin's glands	Usually performed before speculum insertion. Insert index finger into vagina with finger pad upward, and milk urethra and Skene's gland. Note any masses, swelling, discharge, or tenderness.	Area smooth; no swelling, masses, or tenderness.	
Vaginal walls	Note texture, swelling, lesions, or tenderness.	Vaginal wall rugae: no swelling, lesions, nodules, or tenderness. Less rugae in postmenopausal women.	
Perineum	Assess tone and texture.	Perineum smooth, firm in the multiparous woman, thinner in parous woman.	
Cervix	Note size, shape, consistency, position, mobility, or tenderness.	Cervix round, smooth, firm, midline, mobile, and nontender. Cervix smaller in older women. Cervix softer and enlarged during pregnancy.	
Uterus	Note size, shape, symmetry, position, masses, or tenderness.	Uterus midline, may be anteflexed or anteverted, midplane, retroflexed, or retroverted. Pear-shaped, size increases with pregnancy, firm, mobile, slightly tender. No masses.	
Ovaries	Note size, shape, symmetry, or tenderness.	Ovaries usually nonpalpable; if palpable, almond-shaped, firm, smooth, about 3 x 2 x 1 cm, mobile, sensitive to palpation. Ovaries not palpable in postmenopausal women or prepubertal girls.	
Anus and rectum	**Change gloves before rectovaginal exam to prevent cross-contamination.** Perform rectal exam and note sphincter tone, pain, tenderness, nodules, lesions, masses, hemorrhoids, polyps, or bleeding. Note color of stool; **test for occult blood.**	Positive sphincter tone; nontender; no masses, polyps, lesions, hemorrhoids, or bleeding. Stool brown, negative for occult blood.	

(continued)

Assessing the Female Genitourinary System (continued)

Pertinent Health History Findings:

____
____
____
____
____

Pertinent Physical Findings:

____
____
____
____
____

Nursing Diagnoses (Actual or Potential) With Clustered Data:

____
____
____
____
____

Name		Date	
Course		Instructor	

Self-Evaluation Exercise

Female Genitourinary System	Yes	No	Needs More Practice
1. Applies knowledge of anatomy and physiology of the female genitourinary system in performing an assessment of the female genitourinary system.			
2. Applies growth and development principles as applicable to the female genitourinary system.			
3. Considers cultural variations as indicated when performing a female genitourinary assessment.			
4. Gathers all equipment necessary to perform a female genitourinary assessment.			
5. Obtains history specific to assessment of the female genitourinary system.			
6. Performs a physical assessment of the female genitourinary system, including: • General survey and head-to-toe scan. • Inspection. • Palpation. • Pelvic exam.			
7. Documents female genitourinary assessment findings.			
8. Identifies normal/abnormal findings.			
9. Clusters pertinent subjective/objective data.			
10. Identifies actual/potential health problems and states them as nursing diagnoses with supporting data.			

Chapter 19

Assessing the Male Genitourinary System

Name ______________________________ Date ____________

Course ____________________ Instructor ____________________

1. Anatomy review: Label the following structures.
   a. Urinary bladder
   b. Glans penis
   c. Scrotum
   d. Testicle
   e. Ductus deferens
   f. Epididymis
   g. Prostate
   h. Urethra
   i. Rectum
   j. Ampulla of ductus deferens
   k. Seminal vesicle
   l. Corpus cavernosum
   m. Anus
   n. Corpus spongiosum
   o. Bulbourethral gland

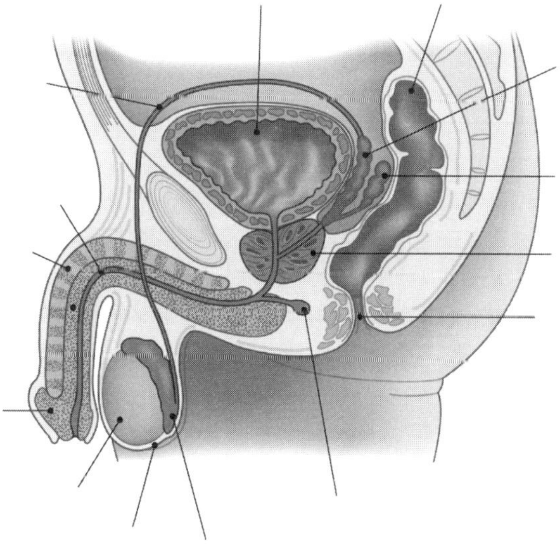

2. Match the structures in the first column to their descriptions in the second column.

Structure	Description
1. Penis	a. Stores sperm until maturity
2. Glans	b. Produces sperm
3. Scrotum	c. Tract for urination
4. Testes	d. Produces alkaline secretions and 20 percent of all semen
5. Vas deferens	e. Protective sheath around the vas deferens
6. Spermatic cord	f. Male organ for copulation and urination
7. Epididymis	g. Tip of penis, sensitive to sexual stimulation
8. Prostate	h. Produce 70 percent of semen
9. Urethra	i. Bulbourethral gland, secretes alkaline secretions
10. Seminal vesicles	j. Sac containing testes, epididymis, and spermatic cord
11. Cowper's gland	k. Muscular tube that holds mature sperm until ejaculation

3. Match the abnormalities in the first column to their descriptions in the second column.

Abnormality	**Description**
1. Tinea cruris	a. Sustained erection
2. Phimosis	b. Urethral opening on dorsal side of penis
3. Priapism	c. "Jock itch" fungal infection
4. Paraphimosis	d. Curved penis
5. Chordee	e. "Bag of worms" varicose veins of spermatic cord
6. Hydrocele	f. Urethral opening on ventral side of penis
7. Varicocele	g. Inflammation of epididymis
8. Spermatocele	h. Lymphatic fluid–filled tunica vaginalis around testis
9. Epididymitis	i. Sperm-filled cyst of epididymis
10. Epispadias	j. Inability to retract foreskin
11. Hypospadias	k. Undescended testicles
12. Cryptorchidism	l. Foreskin retracts but does not return

4. As a high school nurse, you have instituted a testicular self-exam (TSE) program. How would you answer the following questions: Are there any risk factors for testicular cancer? How often should I do a TSE? What do normal testicles feel like?

____

____

____

5. Sam Harrison, age 50, is scheduled for his yearly physical exam, including a prostate screening. At what age should prostate exams begin? What tests are used to screen for prostate cancer?

____

____

6. Mr. Harrison says that he has been having trouble achieving erections. What risk factors might account for this?

____

____

7. The exam should include assessing for hernias. Name three common sites for hernias.

____

____

8. Although your assessment focuses on the male genitourinary system, all systems are related. What assessment findings (subjective or objective) show the relationship between the male genitourinary system and other systems?

____

____

____

Name ______________________________ Date ______________

Course ______________________ Instructor ______________________

Abnormal Case Study: Mike Samuels

Mike Samuels is a 22-year-old college junior. He is on the football team, lives in a residence hall, and does not own a car. He has had six girlfriends during his 3 years at college and has been sexually active with each. Since age 16, he has had gonorrhea once and chlamydia once. He admits that he uses condoms only occasionally. He presents to the clinic saying, "One of my old girlfriends just called me to say that she had a positive human immunodeficiency virus (HIV) test and that I should get checked out."

Health History

CHIEF COMPLAINT:

"One of my old girlfriends just called me to say that she had a positive HIV test and that I should get checked out."

Current Health Status:

Denies any physical symptoms.

Past Health History:

- Had an HIV test 2 years ago as part of his athletic physical. Test results were negative for syphilis and HIV.
- Gonorrhea 5 years ago, treated; return test was negative.
- Chlamydia 3 years ago, treated; did not return for retesting.

9. In this sensitive situation, how would you proceed with the evaluation?

10. From Mr. Samuels' history, identify factors that increase his risk for sexually transmitted diseases (STDs).

11. There are no obvious signs or symptoms to suggest HIV infection. Based on the inspection findings, what other problem would you suspect?

12. Considering Mr. Samuels' assessment findings, what areas should you address for patient education?

Psychosocial Profile:

- *Nutritional patterns:* Usually has healthy appetite, although hasn't been hungry since previous girlfriend contacted him about HIV.
- *Activity/exercise patterns:* Plays on football team.
- *Recreation/hobbies:* No time for hobbies; enjoys dating in spare time, which is usually evenings after studying.
- *Sleep/rest patterns:* Sleeps 5 hours/night.
- *Personal habits:* Smokes marijuana at least once a week, drinks "a lot" of alcohol on the weekends when there is no football game or after the game. Has never used cocaine, barbiturates, narcotics, amphetamines, or intravenous drugs. Has never had a blood transfusion. Has had multiple female sex partners. Has never had sex with another man. Has not knowingly had sex with a prostitute. Engages in sex at least three times a week; occasionally uses condoms.
- *Occupational health patterns:* Student who attends class regularly.
- *Environmental health patterns:* Lives in college residence hall with one roommate. All of his peers have several female friends.

Physical Assessment

- *General appearance:* Healthy 22-year-old man; 6 feet, 1 inch, and 195 lb; keeps head down and makes minimal eye contact; appears anxious.
- *Vital signs:* Normal.
- *Integumentary:*
  - No skin lesions on head, torso, or extremities.
  - Hair evenly distributed; no alopecia.
  - No parasites.
- *Head, eyes, ears, nose, and throat (HEENT):*
  - Oropharynx is pink and moist without lesions.
  - No cervical lymphadenopathy.
- *Penis:*
  - No discharge from penis; multiple wartlike lesions on shaft.
  - No masses felt.
  - No discharge from urethral meatus.
- *Scrotum:*
  - Scrotal skin intact without swelling or lesions. Left is lower than right.
  - No inguinal bulges.
  - Testicles are firm, nontender, and smooth. Epididymis is insensitive to pressure.
- *Inguinal area:*
  - No lymphadenopathy; no palpable masses in inguinal canals bilaterally.

13. Cluster the supporting data for the following nursing diagnoses.

    a. Altered health maintenance related to risky behavior and knowledge deficit of STDs.

    ____

    ____

    b. Risk for infection related to lack of knowledge of disease transmission.

    ____

    ____

    c. Risk for infection transmission related to lack of knowledge of disease transmission.

    ____

    ____

14. Identify any additional nursing diagnoses for Mr. Samuels.

____

____

15. *Word search:* Find the following words in the puzzle: ejaculate, erection, hernia, penis, prostate, scrotum, semen, sperm, testes, urethra.

S	N	O	I	T	C	E	R	E	P
E	C	E	J	A	C	U	T	A	E
H	E	R	N	I	A	S	E	M	N
S	C	R	O	T	U	M	A	C	I
P	R	O	S	T	A	T	E	P	S
E	J	A	C	U	L	A	T	E	U
R	I	N	S	S	E	M	E	N	L
M	U	R	E	T	H	R	A	I	A
P	E	R	S	S	E	T	S	E	T
H	E	R	N	I	S	P	E	R	E

Name ______________________ Date ______________

Course ______________________ Instructor ______________________

Student Lab Sheet: Assessing the Male Genitourinary System

Client's Initials: ______________________

Age: ______________________

Gender: ______________________

Health History

BIOGRAPHICAL DATA:

Current Health Status:
Symptom Analysis (PQRST):

- Pain
- Lesions
- Discharge
- Swelling
- Urinary symptoms
- Erectile dysfunction

Past Health History:

- Childhood illnesses
- Hospitalizations
- Surgeries
- Serious injuries/chronic illness
- Immunizations
- Allergies (food, drugs, environmental)
- Medications (prescribed and over-the-counter [OTC])
- Recent travel/military service

Family History:

Review of Systems:

- General health status
- HEENT
- Respiratory
- Cardiovascular
- Gastrointestinal
- Musculoskeletal
- Neurologic
- Endocrine
- Lymphatic/hematological

Psychosocial Profile:

- Health practices and beliefs/self-care activities
- Typical day
- Nutritional patterns (24-hour recall)
- Activity/exercise patterns
- Recreation, pets, hobbies
- Sleep/rest patterns
- Personal habits (tobacco, alcohol, caffeine, and drugs)
- Occupational health patterns
- Socioeconomic status
- Environmental health patterns
- Roles, relationships, self-concept
- Cultural/religious influences
- Family roles/relationships
- Sexuality patterns
- Social supports
- Stress/coping

Physical Assessment

GENERAL SURVEY:

- Vital signs
- Height
- Weight

Head-to-Toe Scan:

- General health status
- Integumentary
- HEENT
- Respiratory
- Cardiovascular
- Abdominal
- Musculoskeletal
- Neurologic

Assessing the Male Genitourinary System

Area/Physical Assessment Skill	Assessment	Normal Findings Developmental/Cultural Variations	Student's Findings
INSPECTION	**Position: Standing, have patient void before exam.**		
Penis	Inspect dorsal, lateral, and ventral sides. Note condition and color of skin, lesions, and discharge. Note size in relation to physical development and age. Note position of urinary meatus. Note presence of foreskin or circumcision. If uncircumcised, retract foreskin, note ease of retraction and presence of lesions.	Skin intact, color pink to light brown in whites, light to dark brown in African Americans, no lesions or discharge. Urinary meatus midline at tip of glans, foreskin retracts easily.	
Scrotum	Note color, hair distribution, lesions, swelling, size, and position. Note pubic pediculosis.	Skin color darker than rest of body. Hair distribution appropriate for age of patient. Testes hang freely. Left testis slightly lower than right. No lesions, pediculosis.	
Inguinal area	Note condition of skin, bulges. **Have patient bear down and inspect again for any bulges.** Note enlarged lymph nodes.	Skin intact, no bulges, no palpable lymph nodes.	
Rectal area	Note condition of skin, inflammation, rashes, excoriation, rectal prolapse, external hemorrhoids, polyps, lesions, fissures, bleeding, or discharge.	Rectal area intact, no inflammation, lesions, prolapse, hemorrhoids, discharge, or bleeding.	
PALPATION	**Maintain standard precautions, wear gloves.**		
Penis	Note consistency, tenderness, induration, masses, or nodules. Use thumb and two fingers to palpate shaft.	Nonerect penis soft, nontender, no nodules.	

Scrotum, testes, and epididymis	Use thumb and two fingers to palpate surface characteristics of scrotum. Note size, shape, consistency, mobility, masses, nodules, and tenderness of testes. Palpate epididymis and vas deferens on the posterolateral surface, noting swelling or nodules. **Transilluminate any lumps, nodules, or edematous areas.**	Scrotal skin rough without lesions. Testes rubbery, round, movable, smooth, 2 × 5 cm in size, slightly tender with compression. The ridge of epididymis noted and vas deferens smooth and movable. No swelling or nodules.	
Inguinal area	Palpate for inguinal and femoral hernias or masses. **Have patient bear down or cough as you palpate for a bulge or hernia.** Palpate lymph nodes, horizontal and vertical chain. Note enlargement and tenderness.	No inguinal or femoral hernias or masses. No palpable lymph nodes.	
Anus and rectum	**Position: Have patient bend over exam table or lie on side.** Note sphincter tone, pain, tenderness, nodules, lesions, masses, hemorrhoids, polyps, or bleeding. Note color of stool; **test for occult blood.**	Positive sphincter tone, nontender, no masses, polyps, lesions, hemorrhoids, or bleeding. Stool brown; negative for occult blood.	
Prostate	Note size, shape, symmetry, mobility, consistency, nodules, or tenderness.	Prostate walnut shape and size, smooth, rubbery, nontender.	
AUSCULTATION	If scrotal mass detected, auscultate over scrotum for bowel sounds. If present, sign of indirect inguinal hernia.	No bowel sounds.	

(continued)

Assessing the Male Genitourinary System (continued)

Pertinent Health History Findings:

Pertinent Physical Assessment Findings:

Nursing Diagnoses (Actual or Potential) With Clustered Data:

Name		Date	
Course	Instructor		

Self-Evaluation Exercise

Male Genitourinary System	Yes	No	Needs More Practice
1. Applies knowledge of anatomy and physiology of the male genitourinary system in performing an assessment of the male genitourinary system.			
2. Applies growth and development principles as applicable to the male genitourinary system.			
3. Considers cultural variations as indicated when performing a male genitourinary assessment.			
4. Gathers all equipment necessary to perform a male genitourinary assessment.			
5. Obtains history specific to assessment of the male genitourinary system.			
6. Performs a physical assessment of the male genitourinary system, including: • General survey and head-to-toe scan. • Inspection. • Palpation. • Auscultation. • Digital rectal exam.			
7. Documents male genitourinary assessment findings.			
8. Identifies normal/abnormal findings.			
9. Clusters pertinent subjective/objective data.			
10. Identifies actual/potential health problems and states them as nursing diagnoses with supporting data.			

Chapter 20

Assessing the Musculoskeletal System

Name ______________________________ Date ____________

Course ____________________ Instructor ____________________

1. Match the structures in the first column to their descriptions in the second column.

Structure	Description
1. Bursa	a. Allows for upright position and movement; produces heat
2. Tendon	b. Provides structure and support, produces red blood cells, and stores calcium
3. Ligament	c. Connects muscles to bone
4. Cartilage	d. Connects bone to bone
5. Joint	e. Sac filled with synovial fluid that cushions and decreases stress to joints
6. Muscle	f. Articulation of two adjacent bones or cartilage
7. Bone	g. Cushions and absorbs shock

2. What type of synovial joint corresponds to each of the following joints?

   a. Knee ______________________________

   b. Shoulder ______________________________

   c. Wrist ______________________________

   d. Spine ______________________________

   e. Elbow ______________________________

   f. Hip ______________________________

   g. Thumb ______________________________

3. Match the movements in the first column to their descriptions in the second column.

Movement	Description
1. Extension	a. Movement away from midline
2. Flexion	b. Turning inward toward midline
3. Internal rotation	c. Pulling in or backward
4. External rotation	d. Straightening a joint angle
5. Protraction	e. Turning palms up
6. Retraction	f. Turning soles of feet inward
7. Pronation	g. Circular movement
8. Supination	h. Shortening a joint angle
9. Inversion	i. Movement toward the midline
10. Eversion	j. Turning palms down
11. Abduction	k. Turning soles of feet outward
12. Adduction	l. Turning outward away from midline
13. Circumduction	m. Pushing out or forward

4. You are assessing Sarah Parker, a 15-year-old high school sophomore, for scoliosis. You begin by inspecting her spine. What position is best for this?

____

5. As you inspect Sarah's spine, you first note the normal curves. What are the four normal curves of the spine?

____

6. Name and describe the three spinal deformities that you should assess during the spinal exam.

____

____

____

7. Your assessment of Sarah includes leg and arm length measurements. Describe the proper techniques to measure arm lengths and leg lengths.

____

____

8. You note that Sarah's right leg is 2 cm longer than her left leg. Name three findings (subjective or objective) that reflect the effect of the leg-length discrepancy.

____

____

9. You note that Sarah's right upper arm circumference is 1.5 cm greater than her left upper arm circumference. How might you account for this?

____

10. Helen Janewsky, age 70, has degenerative joint disease (DJD) and is 2 days' postoperative after a total right hip replacement. She is ambulating with her walker. You are assessing her gait. What six characteristics should you note?

____

____

11. Name four changes from normal that you would expect to see in Mrs. Janewsky's gait.

____

____

12. What changes in gait might indicate a balance problem?

____

13. Considering Mrs. Janewsky's age, what spinal deformity might you expect to see?

____

14. Because Mrs. Janewsky has DJD, you do a complete assessment of her other joints. Name six characteristics you should note during joint assessment.

____

____

15. You are assessing Mrs. Janewsky's muscle strength. Your findings include: +5 arms, +4 left leg, and +3 right leg. How would you interpret these findings?

____

____

16. Assessment of cerebellar function includes balance, coordination, and accuracy of movement. Name five ways to assess balance.

____

____

17. Name two ways to test coordination of upper and lower extremities.

____

____

18. Name two ways to test accuracy of movements.

____

____

19. Although your assessment focuses on the musculoskeletal system, all systems are related. What assessment findings (subjective or objective) show the relationship between the musculoskeletal system and other systems?

____

____

____

Name ______________________ Date ______________

Course ______________________ Instructor ______________________

Abnormal Case Study: Linda Chu

Linda Chu, a 62-year-old Asian woman, is admitted to the cardiac catheterization unit for a diagnostic procedure to assess coronary artery disease. She is scheduled for the procedure the next morning. She states that she is unable to lie flat for long periods because of chronic low back pain. Because this procedure can take a long time, you need to perform an assessment.

Health History

CHIEF COMPLAINT:

"My lower back hurts all the time."

Symptom Analysis:

P—Pain to lower back when sitting or lying for extended periods.

Q—"Feels like a dull knife in my lower back. I usually get up and walk around to relieve it."

R—"It's my bones; they are getting old."

S—7 on a scale of 1 to 10.

T—Diagnosed with DJD 2 years ago, which has been getting progressively worse.

Current Health Status:

- Pain when sitting or lying for extended periods; 7 on a scale of 1 to 10.
- Stands at her job in a mill pulling cloth through a cutter.
- Takes 4 to 8 ibuprofen tablets (Advil) a day for pain relief.
- Takes lisinopril (Zestril), 5 mg once a day for hypertension (HTN).

Past Health History:

- Normal childhood illnesses.
- Appendectomy at age 8.
- Denies allergies.
- Denies blood transfusions or handicaps.

Family History:

- Family history of HTN.
- Family history of DJD.

Psychosocial Profile:

- *Nutritional patterns:* Eats three balanced meals a day—meat, potatoes, and vegetable. Good milk intake.
- *Recreation/hobbies:* Knits and plays bingo when back isn't hurting too much to sit.
- *Occupational health patterns:* Cutter in a cloth mill. Heavy lifting and pulling are involved in this line of work.
- *Environmental health patterns:* Lives in a two-story home in the country.
- *Roles/relationships:* Lives with husband of 30 years. Has two daughters who visit often. Has not been sexually active for several years because of back problems.

Physical Assessment

- *General appearance:* Stocky appearance: Weight 169 lb; height 5 feet, 4 inches (overweight); position of comfort—two pillows propped behind lower back; facial expression pleasant.
- *Vital signs:* Temperature 98.7°F; pulse 78 beats per minute (BPM); respirations 20/min; blood pressure (BP) 145/78 mm Hg in right arm.
- *Mental status:* Alert and oriented x 3 (person, place, and time).

- *Inspection:*
  - Normal curvature noted to cervical, thoracic, and lumbar spine.
  - Negative deformity noted to cervical, lumbar, and thoracic spine.
- *Palpation:*
  - Negative tenderness to spinous processes.
  - Negative warmth or erythema to spinal processes.

20. What factors increase Mrs. Chu's risk for DJD?

____

21. Aside from Mrs. Chu's history of DJD, what other factors increase her risk for back problems?

____

22. Cluster the supporting data for the following nursing diagnoses:

    a. Pain related to prolonged positions.

    ____

    ____

    ____

    b. Impaired mobility related to pain.

    ____

23. Identify any additional nursing diagnoses for Mrs. Chu.

____

____

24. *Word jumble:* Unscramble the following words. Then unscramble the circled letters to complete the sentence: Two tests for carpal tunnel syndrome are the ____________ and ____________ tests.

    1. (E) N O B
    2. D (T) N E O N
    3. M L (I) G (N) T A E
    4. M (L) U B R A
    5. N (P) I E S
    6. A C L (N) B A E
    7. R S A (L) A C
    8. C I (H) R O T C A
    9. (A) T G I
    10. (E) S L C U M

Name ______________________ Date ____________

Course ______________________ Instructor ______________________

Student Lab Sheet: Assessing the Musculoskeletal System

Client's Initials: ______________________

Age: ______________________

Gender: ______________________

Health History

BIOGRAPHICAL DATA:

Current Health Status:
Symptom Analysis (PQRST):

- Pain
- Weakness
- Deformity
- Activities of daily living (ADL) limitations
- Balance and coordination problems

Past Health History:

- Childhood illnesses
- Hospitalizations
- Surgeries
- Serious injuries/chronic illness
- Immunizations
- Allergies (food, drugs, environmental)
- Medications (prescribed and over-the-counter [OTC])
- Recent travel/military service

Family History:

Review of Systems:

- General health status
- Head, eyes, ears, nose, and throat (HEENT)
- Respiratory
- Cardiovascular
- Gastrointestinal
- Genitourinary
- Neurologic
- Endocrine
- Lymphatic/hematological

Psychosocial Profile:

- Health practices and beliefs/self-care activities
- Typical day
- Nutritional patterns (24-hour recall)
- Activity/exercise patterns
- Recreation, pets, hobbies
- Sleep/rest patterns
- Personal habits (tobacco, alcohol, caffeine, and drugs)
- Occupational health patterns
- Socioeconomic status
- Environmental health patterns
- Roles, relationships, self-concept
- Cultural/religious influences
- Family roles/relationships
- Sexuality patterns
- Social supports
- Stress/coping

Physical Assessment

GENERAL SURVEY:

- Vital signs
- Height
- Weight

Head-to-Toe Scan:

- General health status
- Integumentary
- HEENT
- Respiratory
- Cardiovascular
- Abdominal
- Genitourinary
- Neurologic

Assessing the Musculoskeletal System

Area/Physical Assessment Skill	Assessment	Normal Findings Developmental/Cultural Variations	Student's Findings
INSPECTION	**Positions: Standing, supine, sitting.**		
Posture and spinal curves	Note posture in relation to environment, head position, and body alignment. Note knee position. **Draw an imaginary line from anterior superior iliac crest through knee to feet. Line should transect patella if knees are midline.** Inspect normal curves of spine **(cervical, thoracic, lumbar, and sacral).** If you note spinal deformities, **determine whether they are structural or functional (postural).** Test for kyphosis and scoliosis by having patient bend from waist. Test for lordosis by having patient flatten back against wall.	Posture erect, head midline. Normal spinal curves noted; no kyphosis, scoliosis, or lordosis. Knee aligned with no valgus or varus deviation. **Lordosis is normal in pregnancy and in toddlers.**	
Gait	**Inspect gait as patient walks.** Note wear of shoes. Note phases of gait, arm swing, cadence, base of support, stride length, and toeing. **Wider base of support and shorter stride length often reflects balance problem.**	Phases of gait conform; gait smooth, fluid, and rhythmic; arms swing in opposition; no toeing in or out. Two- to 4-inch base of support, 12- to 14-inch stride length. Shoes worn evenly. Toddlers, elderly, obese, and pregnant patients may have wider base of support, shorter stride length, and uneven rhythm.	
Cerebellar function: Balance	Observe gait, tandem walk (heel to toe), heel-and-toe walk, deep knee bend, Romberg's test. Stand close to patient when performing Romberg's test. Have patient stand with feet together and eyes open, then closed. Swaying is a positive Romberg's test.	Coordinated, balanced gait, positive tandem walk, heel-and-toe walk, deep knee bend. Negative Romberg's test.	
Coordination	Upper extremities: Finger-thumb opposition and rapid alternating movements.	Coordination intact. Rapid alternating movements intact bilaterally. Positive finger-thumb opposition, toe tapping. Able to run heel down shin bilaterally.	

Accuracy of movements	Lower extremities: Toe tapping, running heel down shin. **Note dominant side (usually more coordinated).** Assess point-to-point localization with patient's eyes opened, then closed.	Point-to-point localization intact bilaterally.	
Pronator drift	Test with eyes open, then closed; note drifting.	Negative pronator drift.	
Measurements	Measure arm and leg lengths and circumferences in cm. **Arm length: Measure from acromion process to tip of middle finger.** **Leg length: Measure from anterior superior iliac crest to medial malleolus.** **To ensure accurate circumference measurements, measure at midpoint of extremity.**	Equal arm and leg lengths, or differences that do not exceed 1 cm. Equal arm and leg circumferences, or no more than 1 cm larger on dominant side.	
PALPATION			
Muscle tone	Palpate muscles of upper and lower extremities in relaxed and contracted state. Note any involuntary movement, tenderness, atony, hypotony, or hypertony of muscles.	Muscles at rest soft and pliable, contracted positive muscle tone, firm, no involuntary movements or tenderness.	
Muscle strength	Screen strength with hand grip and foot push/leg raise. Test muscle strength by noting ability to perform active range of motion (ROM) against resistance for face, neck, shoulders, arms, elbows, hands and wrists, hip, knees, ankles, and feet. Grade strength on a 0–5 scale. Compare side to side. **Dominant side may be stronger.**	All muscle groups 4 to 5/5 muscle strength. Hand grip strong and equal; foot push and leg raise against resistance strong and equal.	
INSPECTION/ PALPATION	**Test muscle strength as you assess ROM of joints.**		
Joints	Assess ROM, condition of skin, erythema, edema, heat, deformity, crepitus, tenderness, and stability of all joints.		
Temporo-mandibular joint (TMJ)	Assess as for all joints, with special attention to crepitus or clicks.	Full active ROM (flex, depress, extend, elevate, side to side, protract, and retract). No tenderness, deformity, crepitus, edema, or erythema.	

(continued)

Assessing the Musculoskeletal System (continued)

Area/Physical Assessment Skill	Assessment	Normal Findings Developmental/Cultural Variations	Student's Findings
Cervical spine (neck)	Note cervical curve.	Full active ROM (flex, extend, hyperextend, rotate, lateral bend). No tenderness, crepitus, erythema, or deformity. Normal cervical curve.	
Scapulae	Note location, symmetry, and winging.	Scapula equal over second to seventh rib, no winging.	
Ribs	Note condition of ribs.	Ribs firm, continuous, and nontender.	
Shoulder	Assess as for all joints, with special attention to stability.	Full active ROM (flex, extend, adduct, abduct, internal/external rotate, circumduct). Joint stable; no deformity, crepitus, or tenderness.	
Elbows	Assess as for all joints, with special attention to nodules.	Full active ROM (flex, extend, supinate, pronate). No nodules, crepitus, tenderness, or swelling.	
Wrists	If indicated, assess for carpal tunnel syndrome with Tinel's or Phalen's test.	Full active ROM (flex, extend, hyperextend, radial/ulnar deviation). Joint stable, no crepitus, tenderness. Negative Tinel's and Phalen's tests.	
Fingers and thumbs	Assess as for all joints, with special attention to deformities. Inspect palmar surface for shape and symmetry. Heberden's nodules often on distal interphalangeal joints. Bouchard's nodules often on proximal interphalangeal joints.	Full active ROM (flex, extend, hyperextend, abduct, adduct). Nontender, no deformities. Palms concave and symmetrical.	
Thoracic and lumbar spine	Note thoracic and lumbar curves.	Full active ROM (flex, extend, hyperextend, lateral bends, rotate).	
Hips	Assess as for all joints, with special attention to stability. If indicated, do Trendelenburg's test for hip dislocation. If indicated, do Thomas' test for hip flexure contraction. In newborn, do Ortolani's maneuver to test for hip dislocation. If sciatica present, do straight leg raise	Full active ROM (flex, extend, hyperextend, internal/external rotate, abduct, adduct). Joint stable, no crepitus, nontender.	

Knees	Assess as for all joints, with special attention to crepitus and swelling. If indicated, do McMurray's and Apley's tests for foreign body, torn meniscus. If indicated, do drawer test for anterior cruciate ligament and posterior cruciate ligament tears. If indicated, do bulge sign or patellar tap for fluid.	Full active ROM (flex, extend); knee stable; no swelling, tenderness, crepitus, or nodules.	
Ankles	Assess as for all joints, with special attention to tenderness.	Full active ROM (plantarflex, dorsiflex, evert, invert). No tenderness or crepitus.	
Feet/toes	Assess as for all joints, with special attention to deformities, corns, bunions, hammer toes, and hallux valgus. Note arch, flat feet, or high arches. **Look at type of shoes patient wears. They could be the cause of her or his problems.**	Full active ROM (flex, extend, dorsiflex, abduct, adduct). No deformities; longitudinal arch, weight bearing on foot at midline.	

(continued)

Assessing the Musculoskeletal System (continued)

Pertinent Health History Findings:

Pertinent Physical Assessment Findings:

Nursing Diagnoses (Actual or Potential) With Clustered Data:

Name ______________________________ Date ______________

Course ______________________ Instructor ______________________

Self-Evaluation Exercise

Musculoskeletal System	Yes	No	Needs More Practice
1. Applies knowledge of anatomy and physiology of the musculoskeletal system in performing an assessment of the musculoskeletal system.			
2. Applies growth and development principles as applicable to the musculoskeletal system.			
3. Considers cultural variations as indicated when performing a musculoskeletal assessment.			
4. Gathers all equipment necessary to perform a musculoskeletal assessment.			
5. Obtains history specific to assessment of the musculoskeletal system.			
6. Performs a physical assessment of the musculoskeletal system, including: • General survey and head-to-toe scan. • Inspection. • Palpation.			
7. Documents musculoskeletal assessment findings			
8. Identifies normal/abnormal findings.			
9. Clusters pertinent subjective/objective data.			
10. Identifies actual/potential health problems and states them as nursing diagnoses with supporting data.			

Chapter 21

Assessing the Sensory-Neurologic System

Name ______________________ Date ____________

Course ______________________ Instructor ______________________

1. Anatomy review: Label the following structures.
   a. Frontal lobe
   b. Parietal lobe
   c. Temporal lobe
   d. Occipital lobe
   e. Cerebellum
   f. Lateral fissure
   g. Central fissure
   h. Transversal fissure
   i. Wernicke's area
   j. Broca's area

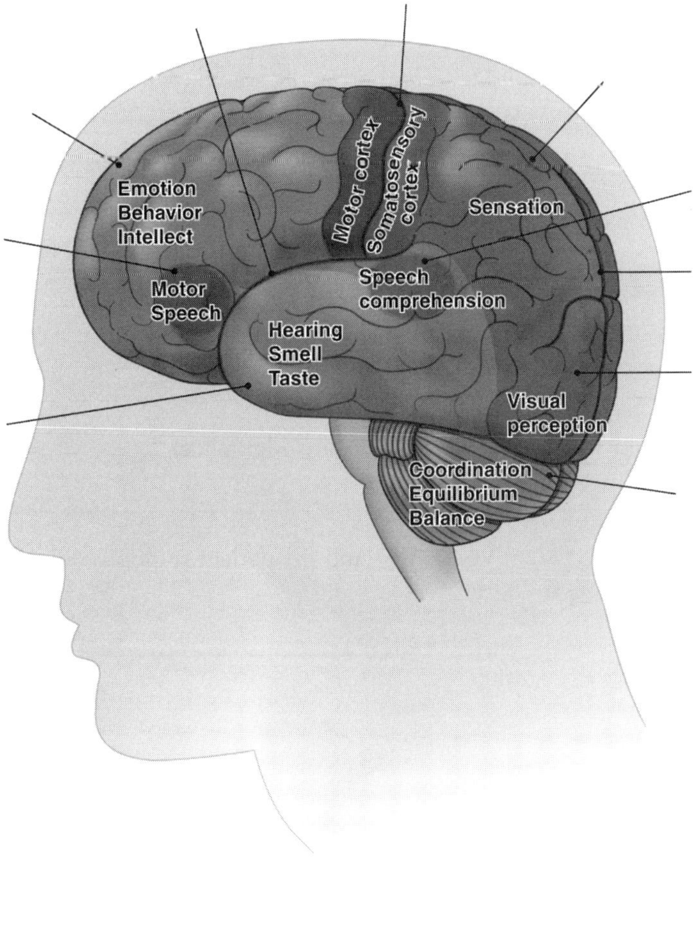

2. Match the neurologic structures in the first column to the appropriate descriptions in the second column.

Structure	Description
1. Cortex	a. Controls balance and coordination of movements
2. Thalamus	b. Controls conscious process
3. Hypothalamus	c. Cardiac and respiratory center
4. Medulla	d. Protective covering of the brain and spine
5. Cerebellum	e. Vision center
6. Temporal lobe	f. Interprets cutaneous sensations
7. Parietal lobe	g. Controls voluntary movement, language expression, and personality
8. Occipital lobe	h. Controls hearing and language comprehension
9. Frontal lobe	i. Maintains consciousness and wakefulness
10. Limbic system	j. Regulates body temperature, appetite, and pituitary hormones
11. Reticular activating system	k. Primitive drives, sexual and emotional arousal
12. Meninges	l. Integrates sensory stimuli

3. Diane Dubrow states that her mother-in-law, Violet, age 77, seems to be getting forgetful. You begin your neurologic assessment of Mrs. Dubrow by assessing her level of consciousness. Name the three areas of orientation you should test.

____

4. If your patient does not respond to verbal or tactile stimuli, what three types of painful stimuli can you use to assess response?

____

5. What two types of painful response should you avoid?

____

6. What three types of memory should you assess to determine memory status?

____

7. What types of memory loss are often seen in the older adult?

____

8. If you ask your patient, "What year is it?" and the patient responds "2050," how would you interpret this response?

____

9. The cranial nerves (CNs) are tested as part of the neurologic exam. Match the cranial nerves in the first column to the appropriate tests in the second column.

Cranial Nerve	Test
1. I: Olfactory	a. Snellen eye chart
2. II: Optic	b. Pupillary reaction
3. III: Oculomotor	c. Smell coffee
4. IV: Trochlear	d. Light touch on face
5. V: Trigeminal	e. Downward eye movement
6. VI: Abducent	f. Taste on anterior portion of tongue
7. VII: Facial	g. Test hearing
8. VIII: Acoustic	h. Taste on posterior portion of tongue
9. IX: Glossopharyngeal	i. Shoulder muscle strength
10. X: Vagus	j. Lateral eye movement
11. XI: Spinoaccessory	k. Range of motion (ROM) of tongue
12. XII: Hypoglossal	l. Gag reflex

10. You also test deep tendon reflexes (DTRs). Match the DTRs in the first column with the appropriate responses in the second column.

Reflex	Response
1. Biceps	a. Knee extension
2. Triceps	b. Flexion at elbow
3. Brachioradialis	c. Plantarflexion
4. Patellar	d. Supination and flexion of wrist
5. Achilles	e. Extension at elbow

11. If you have difficulty eliciting a DTR, what two reinforcement techniques can you use to enhance the response?

____

12. Describe the grading scale that is used to grade the DTR response.

____

____

13. When you assess the plantar reflex, what normal and abnormal responses might you elicit?

____

14. What instructions should you give your patient before performing a sensory exam?

____

15. What sensation can you defer from testing if the patient's pain sensation is intact? Why?

____

____

16. When testing deep and superficial sensations, can you assume that if sensation is intact distally, it is intact in the entire arm?

____

17. Describe the technique for testing vibratory sensation.

____

____

18. Describe the technique for testing kinesthetic sensation.

____

____

19. Match the discriminatory sensations in the first column with the appropriate responses in the second column.

Sensation	Response
1. Graphesthesia	a. Able to identify site that was stimulated
2. Stereognosis	b. Able to identify simultaneous stimuli on opposite sides of body
3. Two-point discrimination	c. Able to identify written number/letter on palm
4. Extinction	d. Able to identify two simultaneous stimuli on skin, closing in until indiscernible
5. Point localization	e. Able to identify object through touch

20. Although your assessment focuses on the sensory-neurologic system, all systems are related. What assessment findings (subjective or objective) show the relationship between the sensory-neurologic system and other systems?

____

____

____

Name ______________________ Date ______________

Course ______________ Instructor ______________________

Abnormal Case Study: Leon Webster

Leon Webster is a 21-year-old, African American college senior. On Friday night, he and several friends went to a local club to celebrate the basketball team's winning season. While driving home, his car hit a tree. He is brought to the ED 30 minutes later by ambulance. Leon is alert and oriented, complaining of a headache and neck pain. He has a 3-inch laceration on his forehead where his head hit the rearview mirror. He was not wearing a seat belt. He was treated in the ED and discharged home with instructions and referral for follow-up.

Three hours later, the patient's mother brings him back to the ED, saying, "Leon says his head really hurts." She states that he cannot keep any food down, that he vomited two times, and that she had a hard time keeping him awake on the ride to the hospital. Because there has been a drastic change in Leon's condition, a focused neurologic assessment is indicated.

Health History

- History of head trauma 5 hours earlier.
- No medication.
- Had been drinking alcohol before accident.
- No history or other neurologic or medical problems.
- No known drug allergies.
- Worsening headache and sleepy.

Physical Assessment

- *General appearance:* Well-groomed; speech clear, but slow; slumped posture; guarding head and neck; sleepy, yet grimacing in pain.
- *Vital signs:* Temperature 98°F; pulse 60 beats per minute (BPM), regular; respirations 20/min; blood pressure (BP) 150/60 mm Hg; pulse oximetry 98 percent room air.
- *Integumentary:* Two-inch sutured laceration on forehead; otherwise negative.
- *Head, eyes, ears, nose, and throat (HEENT):* Facial features symmetrical; pupils 5 mm equal but sluggish reaction.
- *Respiratory:* Lungs clear.
- *Cardiovascular:* Heart sounds 60 BPM and regular, no extra sounds.
- *Abdomen:* Soft, nontender, positive bowel sounds.
- *Musculoskeletal:* +4/5 strength of upper and lower extremities; decreased ROM of neck.
- *Level of consciousness:* Awake, alert, and oriented x 3 but lethargic, falling asleep, Glasgow Coma Scale 14.
- *Communication:* Intact but slow.
- *Memory:* Immediate, remote intact, but doesn't remember events of accident.
- *Cognitive functions*: Too lethargic to test.
- CNs I through XII intact; DTR +2, positive plantar.

21. What may account for the change in Leon's assessment findings?

____

22. What is one of the earliest signs of a change in neurologic status?

____

23. Which of Leon's findings would alert you to a change in intracranial pressure?

____

____

24. Cluster the supporting data for the following nursing diagnoses:

    a. Ineffective cerebral tissue perfusion related to response to injury.

    ____

    ____

    b. Pain related to head and neck trauma.

    ____

    ____

25. Identify any additional nursing diagnoses for Leon.

____

____

____

26. *Word jumble:* Unscramble the following words. Then unscramble the circled letters to complete the sentence: The universal tool used to assess level of consciousness is the _______________.

    1. N B (A) I R
    2. X (C) T R O E
    3. (L) H A S M U T
    4. Y P A (S) N E S
    5. (E) F R A E T N F
    6. (S) R N O U N E
    7. M L B R C E (L) U E E
    8. E L U D M L (A)
    9. E K I (W) R E N C
    10. S A C R B (O) R (A) E A
    11. R Y A (G) R T E T A M
    12. E B M U R E (C)
    13. N (G) I N S E M E
    14. C P T I C (O) I A L B O L E

Name ____________________ Date ____________

Course ____________ Instructor ____________

Student Lab: Assessing the Sensory-Neurologic System

Client's Initials: ____________

Age: ____________

Gender: ____________

Health History

BIOGRAPHICAL DATA:

Current Health Status:
Symptom Analysis (PQRST):

- Headaches
- Dizziness
- Seizures
- Loss of consciousness
- Change in sensation
- Change in mobility
- Dysphagia (difficulty swallowing)
- Dysphasia (difficulty speaking)

Past Health History:

- Childhood illnesses
- Hospitalizations
- Surgeries
- Serious injuries/chronic illness
- Immunizations
- Allergies (food, drugs, environmental)
- Medications (prescribed and over-the-counter [OTC])
- Recent travel/military service

Family History:

Review of Systems:

- General health status
- HEENT
- Respiratory
- Cardiovascular
- Gastrointestinal
- Genitourinary
- Musculoskeletal
- Endocrine
- Lymphatic/hematological

Psychosocial Profile:

- Health practices and beliefs/self-care activities
- Typical day
- Nutritional patterns (24-hour recall)
- Activity/exercise patterns
- Recreation, pets, hobbies
- Sleep/rest patterns
- Personal habits (tobacco, alcohol, caffeine, and drugs)
- Occupational health patterns
- Socioeconomic status
- Environmental health patterns
- Roles, relationships, self-concept
- Cultural/religious influences
- Family roles/relationships
- Sexuality patterns
- Social supports
- Stress/coping

Physical Assessment

GENERAL SURVEY:

- Vital signs
- Height
- Weight

Head-to-Toe Scan:

- General health status
- Integumentary
- HEENT
- Respiratory
- Cardiovascular
- Abdominal
- Genitourinary
- Musculoskeletal

Assessing the Sensory-Neurologic System

Area/Physical Assessment Skill	Assessment	Normal Findings Developmental/Cultural Variations	Student's Findings
	Position: Sitting.		
CEREBRAL FUNCTION	**Consider patient's age, educational and cultural background.**		
Behavior	Note facial expression, posture, affect, and grooming.	Well-groomed, erect posture, pleasant facial expression, appropriate affect. Normal findings vary depending on situation.	
Level of consciousness	Test orientation to time, place, and person. Disorientation to time/place usually occurs before disorientation to person.	Awake, alert, and oriented x 3 (time, place, and person). Older patients may be disoriented to time, but note if they reorient easily.	
Memory	Test immediate, recent, and remote memory. Immediate: Ask patient to repeat a series of numbers. Recent: Name three objects and ask patient to recall them later in exam. Remote: Ask patient his or her birth date and date of major historical event. **If asking for personal data, such as birth date, be sure you can validate information.**	Immediate, recent, and remote memory intact.	
Mathematical/ calculative ability	Have patient perform simple mathematical problem, such as 4 + 5, serial 7s or 4s, subtracting from 100.	Calculative skills intact.	
General knowledge	Assess vocabulary and general knowledge. Ask how many days in a week or months in a year or for definition of familiar words. **Begin with easy words and proceed to more difficult ones (e.g., apple, earthquake, chastise).**	Vocabulary appropriate and general knowledge intact.	
Thought process	Note attention span, logic of speech, ability to stay focused, appropriateness of responses.	Thought process clear, responds appropriately, speech coherent and logical.	
Abstract thinking	Give patient a proverb to interpret. Have patient identify similarities, such as apples and oranges.	Abstract thinking intact.	

Judgment	Assess patient's response to hypothetical situations.	Judgment intact.	
Communication	Note speech and language, enunciation, fluency. Note any dysarthria (difficulty with articulation), dysphasia (difficulty with speech), dysphonia (difficulty/change in voice quality), neologisms (meaningless words), circumlocution (inability to name objects verbally). Test spontaneous speech by having patient describe a picture. Test motor speech by having patient say, "doe, re, mi, fa, so, la, ti, do." Test automatic speech by having patient recite days of week. Test sound recognition by having patient identify familiar sounds. Test auditory-verbal comprehension by noting patient's ability to follow directions. Test visual recognition by having patient identify objects by sight. Test visual-verbal comprehension by having patient read a sentence and explain meaning. Test writing by having patient write name and address. Test copying figures by having patient copy a circle, x, square, triangle, and star. **Start with simple tasks and work to more complex ones.**	Speech clear, fluent; no dysarthria, dysphasia, dysphonia, neologisms, or circumlocution. Communication skills intact: Spontaneous speech, automatic speech, motor speech, sound recognition, auditory-verbal comprehension, visual recognition, visual-verbal comprehension, writing and copying figures.	
CRANIAL NERVES	**Compare side to side.** **Have patient close eyes when testing sensory nerves.**		
CN I—Olfactory	Check patency of nostrils. Test each separately. Note anosmia. Have patient identify a distinct odor (coffee, vanilla).	CN I intact. Sense of smell intact.	

(continued)

Assessing the Sensory-Neurologic System (continued)

Area/Physical Assessment Skill	Assessment	Normal Findings Developmental/Cultural Variations	Student's Findings
CN II—Optic	Test visual acuity, visual fields, retinal structures.	CN II intact. Visual acuity intact.	
CN III—Oculomotor	Test EOM with six cardinal fields, check pupillary reaction to light and accommodation (PERRLA).	CNs III, IV, VI intact. Extraocular muscles intact. OU, PERRLA direct and consensual.	
CN IV—Trochlear			
CN VI—Abducent	If indicated, test oculocephalic reflex. ***Never test oculocephalic reflex (doll's eyes) on a patient with suspected neck injury.***		
CN V—Trigeminal	Test jaw (mastication) muscle strength by having patient bite down on tongue blade. Test sensations on face (forehead, cheeks, chin). Test corneal reflex.	CN V intact. Jaw muscle strength +5, facial sensations intact, positive corneal reflex.	
CN VII—Facial	Test motor function of facial muscles by having patient make faces, smile, frown, and whistle. Test taste (sweet, sour, salty) on anterior portion of tongue.	CN VII intact. Facial movements symmetrical. Taste on anterior tongue intact.	
CN VIII—Acoustic	Test hearing, balance. If indicated, do cold caloric test (oculovestibular reflex) and look for nystagmus (normal response).	CN VIII intact. Hearing and balance intact.	
CNs IX and X—Glossopharyngeal and vagus	Note quality of voice, ability to swallow and cough. Test gag reflex. Look for symmetrical rise of the uvula. Assess taste on posterior third of tongue.	CNs IX and X intact. Strong, clear voice, symmetrical rise of uvula, able to swallow and cough. Positive gag reflex. Taste on posterior tongue intact.	
CN XI—Spinal accessory	Test muscle strength of neck and shoulders.	CN XI intact. +5 muscle strength of neck and shoulders.	
CN XII—Hypoglossal	Test mobility and strength of tongue. Note ability to say "d, l, n, t." Note tongue position, atrophy, or fasciculation.	CN XII intact. Full ROM of tongue, midline, no atrophy or fasciculation.	
SENSORY FUNCTION	**Have patient close eyes. Compare side to side.**		

Light touch, pain, and temperature	Test light touch, pain, and temperature on various areas of body. **If touch sensation intact distally, do not assume it is intact proximally.** **If pain sensation intact, no need to test temperature.** **Avoid using pin because it could break skin. Use sharp and dull sides of toothpick to test pain.**	Light touch, pain, and temperature intact upper and lower extremities.	
Deep sensation: vibratory and kinesthetic (position sense) sensations	Place vibrating tuning fork on bony joint, great toe, and distal interphalangeal joint. Move finger and toe up and down, and have patient identify direction of movement. **If intact distally, intact proximally.**	Vibratory and kinesthetic sensations intact upper and lower extremities.	
Discriminatory sensations:			
Stereognosis	Stereognosis: Have patient identify familiar object (key, paper clip) by touch.	Stereognosis, graphesthesia, two-point discrimination < 5 mm on fingertips, point localization and extinction intact.	
Graphesthesia	Graphesthesia: Draw number or letter in palm of hand and have patient identify.		
Two-point discrimination	Two-point discrimination: Note ability to differentiate being touched at one or two points simultaneously. **Ability to discriminate depends on area tested. Fingertips are most discriminatory.**		
Point localization	Point localization: Note ability to identify a point touched.		
Extinction	Extinction: Note ability to identify two corresponding areas touched simultaneously.		
DEEP TENDON REFLEXES	**Grade DTRs on 0–4 scale.** **If difficulty eliciting reflex, use reinforcement techniques: Clenching teeth, interlocking hands.** **Use percussion hammer.**		
Biceps (C5, C6)	Place your thumb on biceps tendon and strike. Response: Flexion at elbow.	+2/4.	
Triceps (C7, C8)	Strike triceps tendon 1 to 2 inches above elbow. Response: Extension at elbow.	+2/4.	

(continued)

Assessing the Sensory-Neurologic System (continued)

Area/Physical Assessment Skill	Assessment	Normal Findings Developmental/Cultural Variations	Student's Findings
Brachioradialis (C5, C6)	Strike brachioradialis tendon 3 to 5 cm above wrist. Response: Flexion at elbow and supination of hand.	+2/4.	
Patellar (L2, L3, L4)	Strike patellar tendon below patella. Response: Extension of the knees.	+2/4.	
Achilles (S1, S2)	Strike Achilles tendon about 2 inches above heel. Response: Plantar-flexion of the foot.	+2/4.	
SUPERFICIAL REFLEXES	**Grade as positive or negative.**		
Plantar (L4 to S2)	Stroke sole of foot from heel laterally across ball of foot to great toe. Response: Flexion of toes. **Babinski response: Dorsiflexion of great toe and fanning of toes.**	Positive plantar reflex. Babinski normal in infants.	
Abdominal (T8, T9, T10)	Stroke each quadrant of abdomen toward umbilicus. Response: Umbilicus moves toward stimulus.	Positive abdominal reflex. May be absent in obese or pregnant patients.	
Anal (S3, S4, S5)	Scratch side of anus. Response: Puckering of anus.	Positive anal reflex.	
Cremasteric (L1, L2)	Stroke inner aspect of male's thigh. Response: Elevation of testes.	Positive cremasteric reflex.	
Bulbocavernous (S3, S4)	Gently apply pressure over bulbocavernous muscle and gently pinch foreskin or glans. Response: Contraction of bulbocavernous muscle.	Positive bulbocavernous reflex.	

Pertinent Health History Findings:

Pertinent Physical Assessment Findings:

Nursing Diagnoses (Actual or Potential) With Clustered Data:

Name ____________________ Date ____________

Course ____________________ Instructor ____________________

Self-Evaluation Exercise

Sensory-Neurologic System	Yes	No	Needs More Practice
1. Applies knowledge of anatomy and physiology of the sensory-neurologic system in performing an assessment of the sensory-neurologic system.			
2. Applies growth and development principles as applicable to the sensory-neurologic system.			
3. Considers cultural variations as indicated when performing a sensory-neurologic assessment.			
4. Gathers all equipment necessary to perform a sensory-neurologic assessment.			
5. Obtains history specific to assessment of the sensory-neurologic system.			
6. Perform a physical assessment of the sensory-neurologic system, including: • General survey and head-to-toe scan. • Inspection. • Palpation. • Reflexes.			
7. Documents sensory-neurologic assessment findings.			
8. Identifies normal/abnormal findings.			
9. Clusters pertinent subjective/objective data.			
10. Identifies actual/potential health problems and states them as nursing diagnoses with supporting data.			

Chapter 22

Putting It All Together

Name ______________________ Date ____________

Course ______________________ Instructor ______________________

Sample Assessment Form

Health History

BIOGRAPHICAL DATA:

Name: ______________________

Address: ______________________

Phone number: ______________________

Contact person (relationship to patient): ______________________

Age: ______________________ Marital status: ______________________

Birth date: ______________________ Number of dependents: ______________________

Birthplace: ______________________ Educational level: ______________________

Gender: ______________________ Occupation: ______________________

Ethnicity/nationality: ______________________ Advance directive: ______________________

Social Security number: ______________________ Health insurance: ______________________

Referral (primary care physician/practitioner): ______________________

Source of history/reliability: ______________________

Reason for Seeking Healthcare:

____

____

Past Health History:

Childhood illnesses: ______________________

Hospitalizations: ______________________

Surgeries: ______________________

Serious injuries/chronic illnesses: ______

Immunizations: ______

Allergies (food, drugs, environmental): ______

Medications (prescribed/over-the-counter [OTC]): ______

Recent travel/military service: ______

FAMILY HISTORY:

______

______

Review of Systems:

General health status: ______

Integumentary: ______

Skin: ______

Hair: ______

Nails: ______

Head, eyes, ears, nose, throat (HEENT): ______

Head and neck: ______

Eyes: ______

Ears: ______

Nose and sinuses: ______

Mouth and throat: ______

Respiratory: ______

Cardiovascular: ______

Breasts: ______

Gastrointestinal: ______

Genitourinary: ______

Female/male reproductive: ______

Musculoskeletal: ______

Neurologic: ______

Endocrine: ______

Immune/hematological: ______

Developmental:

______

______

Psychosocial Profile:

Health practices and beliefs/self-care activities: ______

Typical day: ______

Nutritional patterns (24-hour recall): ____________________

Activity/exercise patterns: ____________________

Recreation, pets, hobbies: ____________________

Sleep/rest patterns: ____________________

Personal habits (tobacco, alcohol, caffeine, and drugs): ____________________

Occupational health patterns: ____________________

Socioeconomic status: ____________________

Environmental health patterns: ____________________

Roles, relationships, self-concept: ____________________

Cultural/religious influences: ____________________

Family roles/relationships: ____________________

Sexuality patterns: ____________________

Social supports: ____________________

Stress/coping patterns: ____________________

Summary of Pertinent Health History Findings:

____

____

Physical Assessment

GENERAL APPEARANCE:

Vital signs: Temperature ____________________; pulse ____________________; respirations ____________________; blood pressure (BP) (left/right) ____________________

Height: ____________________

Weight: ____________________

Integumentary: ____________________

HEENT: ____________________

Head and neck: ____________________

Eyes: ____________________

Ears: ____________________

Nose and sinuses: ____________________

Mouth and throat: ____________________

Respiratory: ____________________

Cardiovascular: ____________________

Breasts: ____________________

Abdomen: ____________________

Female/male reproductive: ____________________

Musculoskeletal: ____

Neurologic: ____

Endocrine: ____

Lymphatic/hematological: ____

Summary of Pertinent Physical Assessment Findings:

____

____

Name ______________________ Date ____________

Course ______________________ Instructor ______________________

Assessment Form "Guide at a Glance"

Health History

BIOGRAPHICAL DATA:

Name: ______________________

Address: ______________________

Phone number: ______________________

Contact person (relationship to patient): ______________________

Age: ____________ Marital status: ____________

Birth date: ____________ Number of dependents: ____________

Birthplace: ____________ Educational level: ____________

Gender: ____________ Occupation: ____________

Ethnicity/nationality: ____________ Advance directive: ____________

Social Security number: ____________ Health insurance: ____________

Referral (primary care physician/practitioner): ______________________

Source of history/reliability: ______________________

REASON FOR SEEKING HEALTHCARE:

Primary level: Include usual state of health, any major health problems, usual patterns of healthcare, and health concerns.

Secondary and tertiary levels: Identify chief complaint and do symptom analysis (PQRST).

PAST HEALTH HISTORY

Childhood illnesses: Ask about mumps, chickenpox, rubella, ear infections, streptococcal infections or sore throats, scarlet fever, pertussis, and asthma.

Hospitalizations: Include name of hospital, reason for hospitalization, physician name, dates, and length of stay.

Surgeries: Include surgical procedures, physician name, and hospital.

Serious injuries: Include head injuries with loss of consciousness, fractures, motor vehicle accidents, burns, and lacerations.

Chronic illnesses: Include heart disease, hypertension (HTN), diabetes, cancer, and seizures.

Immunizations: Age dependent; include measles, mumps, rubella, tetanus, diphtheria, pertussis, chickenpox, hepatitis B, polio, *Haemophilus influenzae* B (HIB), pneumococcal vaccine, influenza, meningitis, tuberculosis testing.

Allergies: Include food, drug, and environmental allergens and whether patient ever had penicillin. If positive for allergy, state type of reaction.

Medications: Include prescribed and OTC, including vitamin and herbal supplements. Assess patient's understanding of medications.

Recent travel/military service: Include travel within past year and recent and past military service.

FAMILY HISTORY

Include patient, spouse, children, parents, siblings, aunts, uncles, and grandparents. List family members or draw a genogram.

REVIEW OF SYSTEMS

General health status: Ask about fatigue, exercise intolerance, unexplained fever, night sweats, weakness, difficulty with activities of daily living (ADL), and number of colds and illnesses per year.

Integumentary:

Skin: Ask about skin diseases, itching, rashes, scars, sores, ulcers, warts, moles, changes in skin lesions, and skin reactions to hot and cold. Ask about piercings and tattoos.

Hair: Ask about changes in hair texture, baldness, unusual patterns, and hair care (e.g., shampoo, coloring, permanents).

Nails: Ask about changes in nails, color, texture, splitting, cracking, and nail care (e.g., use of polish or acrylic nails).

HEENT:

Head and neck: Ask about headaches, lumps, scars, recent head trauma, injury or surgery, history of concussion, loss of consciousness, dizzy spells, fainting, stiff neck, pain with head movement, swollen glands, and nodes or masses.

Eyes: Ask about use of corrective lenses (glasses or contact lenses), visual deficits, last eye exam, last glaucoma check, eye injury, itching, tearing, drainage, pain, floaters, halos, loss of vision of parts of fields, blurred vision, double vision, colored lights, flashing lights, light sensitivity, twitching, cataracts, glaucoma, eye surgery, retinal detachment, strabismus, and amblyopia.

Ears: Ask about last hearing test, difficulty hearing, sensitivity to sounds, ear pain, drainage, vertigo, ear infections, ringing, fullness, wax problems, use of hearing aids, ear care habits and ear piercings.

Nose and sinuses: Ask about nosebleeds, broken nose, deviated septum, snoring, postnasal drip, runny nose, sneezing, allergies, use of recreational drugs, difficulty breathing through nose, problem with ability to smell, pain over sinuses, sinus infections.

Mouth and throat: Ask about sore throats, streptococcal infections, mouth sores, oral herpes, bleeding gums, hoarseness, changes in quality of voice, difficulty chewing or swallowing, changes in sense of taste, dentures and bridges, dental health and hygiene patterns, tongue piercings, dental surgery, and date of last dental exam.

Respiratory: Ask about breathing problems, cough, sputum (color and amount), shortness of breath with activity, noisy respirations, pneumonia, tuberculosis, bronchitis, last chest x-ray, purified protein derivative (PPD) and results, and history of smoking.

Cardiovascular: Ask about chest pain, palpitations, murmurs, skipped beats, HTN, awakening at night, shortness of breath, dizzy spells, cold or numb hands and feet, color changes in hands and feet, swelling of extremities, hair loss on legs, sores that do not heal, and electrocardiograms (ECGs) and results.

Breasts: Ask about breast masses, lumps, pain, discharge, swelling, changes in breasts or nipples, cystic breast disease, breast cancer, breast surgery, reduction/enhancement, breast self-exam (BSE; when and how), date of last clinical breast exam, and mammograms and results.

Gastrointestinal: Ask about appetite and changes, indigestion, heartburn, gastroesophageal reflux disease, nausea, vomiting, vomiting blood, liver or gallbladder disease, jaundice, abdominal swelling, bowel patterns and changes, color and consistency of stools, diarrhea, constipation, hemorrhoids, weight changes, use of laxatives, antacids, date and results of last fecal occult blood test, and colonoscopies and results.

Genitourinary: Ask about pain on urination, burning, frequency, urgency, dribbling, incontinence, hesitancy, changes in urine stream, color of urine, history of urinary tract infections, kidney infections, kidney disease, kidney stones, and frequent nighttime urination.

Female/male reproductive: *Female*: Ask about menarche, description of cycle, last menstrual period (LMP), painful menses, excessive bleeding, irregular menses, bleeding between periods, last Pap test and results, satisfaction with sexual performance, painful intercourse, use of contraceptives, sexually transmitted diseases (STDs), knowledge of STD prevention, safe sex practices, infertility problems, pregnancies, live births, miscarriages, and abortions. *Male*: Ask about lesions, discharge, pain on urination, painful intercourse, prostate or scrotal problems, history of STDs, knowledge of STD prevention, safe sex practices, infertility problems, impotence or sterility, satisfaction with sexual performance, frequency and technique for testicular self-exam (TSE), and last prostate exam and results.

Musculoskeletal: Ask about fractures, sprains, muscle cramps, pain, weakness, joint swelling, redness, limited range of motion (ROM), joint deformity, noise with movement, spinal deformities, low back pain, loss of height, osteoporosis, degenerative joint disease (DJD), rheumatoid arthritis, use of calcium supplements, ability to do ADL, and bone density scan and results.

Neurologic: Ask about loss of consciousness; fainting; seizures; head injury; changes in cognition; memory; hallucinations; disorientation; speech problems; sensory deficits such as numbness, tingling, and loss of sensation; motor problems; problems with gait, balance, and coordination; and ability to do ADL.

Endocrine: Ask about thyroid disease; diabetes; changes in weight, thirst, hunger, or urination; heat and cold intolerance; goiter; weakness; hormone therapy; and changes in skin and hair.

Lymphatic/hematological: Ask about bleeding disorders, recurrent infections, cancers, human immunodeficiency virus (HIV), fatigue, blood transfusions, bruising, allergies, and unexplained swollen nodes.

Developmental: Identify current developmental level and prior developmental problems.

PSYCHOSOCIAL PROFILE

Health practices and beliefs/self-care activities: Ask about perceived health, what patient does to stay healthy, yearly physical exams, self-exams.

Typical day: Ask about usual day from time patient awakens until bedtime.

Nutritional patterns: Do a 24-hour recall and compare with food groups. Use weekday diet.

Activity/exercise patterns: Ask about types and amounts of exercise and use of protective equipment.

Recreation, pets, hobbies: Identify health risk factors.

Sleep/rest patterns: Ask about number of hours of sleep per night, whether sleep is restful, naps, and use of sleep aids.

Personal habits (tobacco, alcohol, caffeine, and drugs): Ask about type, amount, and years used.

Occupational health patterns: Identify health risks or exposure to toxic substances.

Socioeconomic status: Ask about health insurance.

Environmental health patterns: Identify environment as urban/rural; ask about safety of home and neighborhood, type of home, heating and plumbing, and smoke detectors.

Roles, relationships, self-concept: Ask about roles/relationships and how patient sees self.

Cultural/religious influences: Identify cultural and religious influences on health.

Family roles/relationships: Identify patient's role in family and number of dependents in family.

Sexuality patterns: Identify sexual patterns, preferences, and safe sex practices.

Social supports: Identify supports, family, friends, coworkers, and community agencies.

Stress/coping patterns: Identify amount of stress and coping mechanisms.

Physical Assessment

HEAD-TO-TOE PHYSICAL ASSESSMENT: GENERAL SURVEY

General appearance: Include age, general appearance, grooming, hygiene, odors, nutritional status, level of consciousness, speech, affect, gait, posture, movements, gross deformities, and signs of distress.

Vital signs: Temperature ____________________;

pulse __________; respirations ________________;

BP (left/right) ______________ Height: ________

Weight: ____________________________________

Integumentary: Inspect color and lesions and palpate temperature, turgor, and texture throughout exam.

HEENT

Head: Inspect size, shape and symmetry, position, hair distribution, and lesions; palpate scalp mobility, tenderness, and hair texture.

Face: Inspect symmetry of nasolabial folds and palpebral fissures; palpate temporal arteries and temporomandibular joint (TMJ); test ROM; and test facial sensations (cranial nerve [CN] V), facial expressions, and ability to smile and frown (CN VII).

Eyes: Test visual acuity near/far with Snellen chart (CN II), color vision, peripheral vision by confrontation, extraocular movement in six cardinal fields (CNs III, IV, and VI), and corneal light reflex; perform cover-uncover test; test corneal blink reflex; inspect external structures (general appearance of eyes, lids, sclera, conjunctiva, cornea, lens, and anterior chamber of the iris); palpate lacrimal glands and ducts; test pupils; and perform funduscopic examination of disc, arteries and veins, fundus, and macula.

Ears: Inspect/palpate external ear; check angle of attachment; perform Weber, Rinne, and whisper tests (CN VIII); and perform otoscopic exam of canal and tympanic membrane.

Nose and sinuses: Palpate sinuses for tenderness and nasal patency; test sense of smell (CN I); and inspect nasal mucosa, septum, and turbinates.

Mouth: Inspect/palpate lips, oral mucosa, teeth, and gingiva; inspect tongue; test taste on anterior/posterior tongue (CNs VII, IX); test mobility of tongue (CN XII); test gag/swallow reflex (CNs IX, X); and palpate parotid and submandibular glands.

Neck: Inspect, palpate, and auscultate thyroid gland; palpate and auscultate carotids; measure jugular venous pressure; palpate nodes and tracheal position; note ROM of neck; and test neck muscle strength (CN XI).

Posterior thorax/lungs: Palpate excursion and fremitus, percuss lungs and diaphragmatic excursion, and auscultate breath sounds.

Posterior thorax/spine: Inspect normal spinal curves; test for scoliosis, kyphosis, and lordosis; check ROM of spine; palpate paravertebral muscles for tenderness; fist/blunt percuss costovertebral angle tenderness.

Anterior thorax/breast: Inspect and palpate breast and lymph nodes with patient in various positions.

Anterior thorax/lungs: Inspect anteroposterior: lateral ratio, palpate excursion and fremitus, percuss chest, and auscultate breath sounds.

Anterior thorax/heart: Inspect and palpate precordium for pulsations, note point of maximal impulse (PMI), and auscultate heart sounds.

Upper extremities: Palpate brachial, radial, and ulnar pulses; perform Allen's test if indicated; perform Tinel's or Phalen's test for carpal tunnel syndrome if indicated; check color, temperature, capillary refill, deformities, and clubbing of hands and nails; inspect joints for deformities; test hand grip; check ROM and strength; measure arm length and circumferences; test pronator drift; test coordination with rapid alternating movements and finger-thumb opposition; test accuracy of movements with point-to-point localization; test superficial and deep sensations; and test deep tendon reflex (DTR) of upper extremities.

Abdomen: Inspect size, shape, symmetry, and movements (respirations, pulsations, and peristalsis); test for hernias; auscultate bowel and vascular sounds; percuss abdomen and organs; if ascites suspected, percuss for shifting dullness; and palpate abdominal organs (liver, kidneys, and spleen), aorta, inguinal lymph nodes, and femoral arteries.

Lower extremities: Inspect color, hair distribution, and varicose veins; perform Trendelenburg test or manual compression test to check venous circulation, if indicated; palpate pedal pulses and temperature; inspect condition of feet and toenails and note lesions and deformities; test ROM of lower extremities; measure leg lengths and circumferences; perform straight leg test if indicated; perform patellar tap or bulge sign if fluid suspected; check for drawer sign if torn anterior cruciate ligament or posterior cruciate ligament suspected; perform Apley's or McMurray's test if meniscus tear suspected; test muscle strength and superficial and deep sensations; inspect gait, toe-and-heel walking, tandem walk, and deep knee bend; perform Romberg's test; have patient toe tap and run heel down shin; and test Achilles, patellar DTR, and plantar reflexes.

Female genitalia/rectum: Inspect and palpate external and internal genitalia, obtain specimens as indicated, inspect and palpate inguinal nodes and rectum for masses, and test stool for occult blood.

Male genitalia/rectum: Inspect and palpate male genitalia, inspect and palpate inguinal nodes and rectum for masses, and test stool for occult blood. Palpate prostate and check for hernias.

USING THE FOUR TECHNIQUES OF PHYSICAL ASSESSMENT BY SYSTEM

Integumentary:

Skin:

Inspect: Color, lesions (note location, distribution, configuration, and morphology), and vascular lesions.

Palpate: Moisture, temperature, texture, elasticity (turgor), and masses.

Hair:

Inspect: Color and distribution.

Palpate: Texture.

Nails:

Inspect: Color, angle of attachment, and markings.

Palpate: Texture and capillary refill.

HEENT:

Head and face:

Inspect: Size, shape, symmetry, nasolabial folds, palpebral fissures, edema, pigmentation, lesions, tics, and grimacing.

Palpate: Skull and mobility of scalp.

Neck:

Inspect: Three positions (neutral, hyperextended, and as patient swallows), anterior and posterior triangles, and trachea.

Palpate: Trachea, lymph nodes, and thyroid.

Eyes:

Test visual acuity: Near/far vision, peripheral vision, color vision, position and alignment of extraocular muscles, corneal light reflex, six cardinal fields, and cover-uncover test.

Inspect: General appearance, lashes, lids, conjunctiva, sclera, cornea, anterior chamber, iris, and pupils.

Palpate: Lacrimal glands and ducts.

Funduscopic: Vessels, disc, retina, and macula.

Ears:

Test hearing: Whispered voice sounds, Weber test, and Rinne test.

Inspect: Angle of attachment, position and drainage, and shape and symmetry.

Palpate: Consistency, nodules, tragus, mastoid, and pull helix forward.

Otoscopic examination: External ear canal: color, patency, drainage; tympanic membrane: color, drainage, landmarks, intactness, and mobility of drum.

Nose:

Inspect: Position, drainage, septal deviation, nasal mucosa, and turbinates.

Palpate: Nasal patency and tenderness.

Sinuses:

Inspect: Edema.

Palpate: Tenderness.

Percuss: Tenderness.

Transilluminate: Fluid.

Mouth and throat:

Inspect: Note odor of breath.

Lips: Color, lesions, hydration. *Teeth:* Number, condition, color, and occlusion. *Gingivae:* Color, bleeding, and retraction or hypertrophy. *Oral mucosa:* Color, lesions. *Tongue:* Color, hydration, mobility, Stensen's and Wharton's ducts, patency, and inflammation. *Tonsils:* Color, size, and exudates. *Palates*: Color and intactness. *Uvula*: Position and symmetry. *Pharynx*: Color and exudates.

Palpate: Parotid, submandibular, and sublingual glands.

Respiratory:

Inspect: Respirations, rate, rhythm, size, shape, symmetry, anteroposterior:lateral ratio, excursion, muscles of breathing, and condition of skin.

Palpate: Chest for tenderness, crepitus, tactile fremitus, and excursion.

Percuss: Chest for resonance and diaphragmatic excursion.

Auscultate: Breath sounds (vesicular, bronchovesicular, and bronchial), abnormal sounds, adventitious sounds, and abnormal voice sounds.

Cardiovascular:

Inspect: Neck vein distension, pulsations on neck and precordium, measure jugular venous pressure.

Palpate: Pulses: rate, rhythm, equality, amplitude, contour and elasticity, and thrills; precordial sites for pulsations, thrills, lifts, and heaves.

Percuss: Cardiac borders.

Auscultate: Normal heart sounds (intensity, pitch, timing in cardiac cycle, location, and splits), extra sounds OS, ejection click, S_3, S_4, murmurs and rubs, bruits, and venous hums.

Breasts:

Inspect: Positions (sitting hands at side, hands pressed on hips, hands over head, leaning forward, and supine with small pillow under shoulder of breast being examined), size, shape, symmetry, color, condition of skin, lesions, venous pattern, dimpling, retraction, masses, nipple position, inverted/everted, discharge, and axilla (color, rashes, and masses).

Palpate: Three levels (light, medium, and deep pressure), consistency, masses, tenderness, nipples for discharge, and lymph node enlargement.

Abdomen:

Inspect: Size, shape, symmetry, movements (respiratory, pulsations, and peristalsis), hernias, skin condition, venous pattern lesions, and umbilicus color and position (inverted or everted).

Auscultate: Bowel sounds, vascular sounds and rubs; scratch test.

Palpate: Light: surface characteristics; Deep: abdominal organs (liver, spleen, and kidneys), rebound tenderness, rigidity, and aortic pulsation and size.

Percuss: Abdomen, liver, spleen, and kidneys for costovertebral angle tenderness; bladder for distension; and shifting dullness if ascites.

Female/male reproductive:

Female:

Inspect: External genitalia, vaginal mucosa, and cervix.

Palpate: Vaginal wall, cervix, uterus, adnexa, and rectum.

Obtain: Specimens as indicated.

Male:

Inspect: External genitalia, penis and scrotum, and inguinal area.

Palpate: Penis, scrotum and testes, inguinal hernias, inguinal nodes, rectum, and prostate.

Obtain: Specimens as indicated.

Musculoskeletal:

Inspect: Posture, gait, spinal curves (cervical, thoracic, lumbar, and sacral), joints (condition of skin, deformities, stability, crepitus, erythema, and ROM), cerebellar function (balance, coordination, and accuracy of movements), and limb measurements.

Palpate: Muscle tone, strength, joint deformities, tenderness, and heat.

Percuss: Patella for fluid.

Neurologic:

Test:

Cerebral function: Level of consciousness, memory, communication, mental status, thought process, affect, judgment, vocabulary, and calculation.

Cranial nerves: CNs I through XII.

Sensory: Superficial: light touch, pain, temperature; Deep: vibratory, kinesthetic, graphesthesia, stereognosis, two-point discrimination, extinction, and point localization.

DTRs: Biceps, triceps, brachioradialis, patellar, and Achilles (grade 0–4).

Superficial reflexes: Plantar, abdominal, cremasteric, and bulbocavernosus.

Summary of Pertinent Physical Assessment Findings:

____

____

Name ______________________ Date ______________

Course ______________________ Instructor ______________________

Abnormal Case Study: Harry Holsvick

Harry Holsvick is a 32-year-old, white, male construction worker with two children. You are seeing him in the clinic for a health risk assessment.

Health History

BIOGRAPHICAL DATA:

- Construction worker.
- Married with two children (ages 2 and 5).
- Roman Catholic.

Current Health Status:

- No current health problems.
- No known drug, environmental, or food allergies.
- Concerned about his father's recent heart attack and his own future heath risks.
- Seeks a health risk screening.
- No current prescription medications. Occasionally uses OTC medications for colds or headaches and takes ibuprofen for work-related aches and pains about 2 days per week.

Past Health History:

- No history of medical problems.
- Had chickenpox as a child.
- Leg laceration last year from falling piece of construction equipment. Healed with no complications.
- Had all childhood immunizations. Most recent tetanus last year after leg injury. Cannot remember if he had a PPD.
- No surgeries. Was hospitalized once as a teenager after a football injury when he lost consciousness for several minutes. Has been to the ED twice in past 5 years for injuries suffered on the job.

Family History:

- Mother, age 64, alive and well.
- Father, age 67, HTN and recent myocardial infarction.
- Sisters, ages 27 and 34, alive and well.
- Maternal grandmother, age 85, HTN.
- Maternal grandfather, died of myocardial infarction at age 81.
- Maternal aunt, age 60, alive and well.
- Maternal uncle, age 66, HTN.
- Paternal grandmother, age 87, HTN, stroke.
- Paternal grandfather, died of myocardial infarction at age 85.
- Paternal aunt, age 68, HTN.
- Paternal uncle, age 65, HTN.
- Denies family history of diabetes, kidney disease, allergies, asthma, drug or alcohol addiction, tuberculosis, bleeding disorders, or mental disorders.

Review of Systems:

- **General health status:** No fever, chills, fatigue, depression, anxiety, or weight gain or loss this year. Says overall health is good. Weight has been stable for the last 5 years.
- **Integumentary:** No rashes, lesions, mole changes, or bruising.
- **HEENT:** No headaches, vision problems, hearing problems, sinus problems, frequent sore throats, or hoarseness.
- **Respiratory:** No shortness of breath, wheezing, cough, productive cough, or history of tuberculosis.
- **Cardiovascular:** No history of HTN, heart problems or murmurs, blood clots/phlebitis, chest pain, palpitations, edema, orthopnea, or claudication.

- **Gastrointestinal:** No nausea/vomiting, abdominal pain, dysphagia, heartburn, jaundice, hemorrhoids, or blood in stool.
- **Genitourinary:** No dysuria, frequency, urgency, penile discharge, or testicular masses; satisfied with sex life.
- **Musculoskeletal:** No joint pains, swelling, or muscle weakness.
- **Neurologic:** No dizziness, vertigo, syncope, seizures, or numbness or tingling of extremities. History of a concussion in high school. Has never been treated for a mental disorder, depression, or anxiety.
- **Endocrine:** No polyuria/polydipsia or heat or cold intolerance.
- **Lymphatic/hematological:** No known exposure to hepatitis or other infectious disease; no cancer, bleeding, or anemia; has not had a blood transfusion.

Psychosocial Profile:

- **Self-care activities:** Does not seek routine healthcare screenings and has not had a physical exam in 2 years. Feels he is healthy and does not need to seek care unless he is sick or injured. Does not know his cholesterol level or usual BP. Does not know how to do TSE.
- **Typical day:** Arises at 4:30 A.M. Commutes to work and begins at 7:00 A.M. and works until 3:30 P.M. Drives home and relaxes, watches the news, and spends time with his family. He goes to bed by 10:00 P.M. each night.
- **Nutritional patterns:** Feels he eats a balanced diet, but evaluation reveals it is high in fats and cholesterol. Weight has been stable for last 5 years. 24-hour recall: Breakfast—8 oz coffee with cream and 2 tsp sugar, 4 oz orange juice, cream-filled donut. Lunch—Cheesesteak sandwich, French fries, and soda. Dinner—Fried chicken, mashed potatoes with butter, peas, salad with blue cheese dressing, 8 oz glass of milk, and 8 oz coffee with cream and 2 tsp of sugar, chocolate ice cream. Snack—Four chocolate chip cookies.
- **Activity/exercise patterns:** Work requires vigorous physical activity, including stair climbing, lifting, and repetitive motions. Sometimes plays basketball with friends on weekends.
- **Recreation/hobbies:** Enjoys watching sports on TV and taking camping trips.
- **Sleep/rest patterns:** Sleeps well 7 to 8 hours a night and feels rested in the morning. Sometimes falls asleep watching television after dinner.
- **Personal habits:** Has six beers each weekend when watching sports programs. Has smoked five to eight cigarettes a day for the last 10 years. Denies recreational drug use.
- **Occupational health patterns:** States there are risks at work, but he takes full advantage of safety measures available.
- **Roles/relationships:** States he is in a good marriage that is supportive. States he is comfortable with his sexual relationship with his wife. Enjoys his children, especially his 5-year-old son.
- **Stress and coping:** Copes with problems by discussing them with wife. Often tries not to think about things that bother him.
- **Environmental health patterns:** Commute varies depending on location of current job, but is usually 30 to 50 miles/day. Usually wears seatbelt in car.

1. What would you include in Mr. Holsvick's physical assessment based on information provided in the health history?

____

2. What health education does the patient need for his age, sex, and health risks?

____

____

Physical Assessment Findings

- **General appearance:** A 32-year-old, well-developed, well-nourished, white man who appears stated age; no apparent distress at this time; moves all extremities well, gait normal. Dressed in work clothes and dusty.
- **Vital signs:** Temperature 97.9°F; pulse 68 beats per minute (BPM); respirations 20/min; BP 138/86 mm Hg; height 5 feet, 9 inches; weight 170 lb.
- **Mental status:** Oriented to person, place, and time; appropriate affect; language well developed.
- **Integumentary**
  - Skin evenly colored, dry, without any worrisome lesions.
  - Scar from work injury present on left lower leg.
  - Hands dry with abrasions.
  - Hair clean and thin.
  - No clubbing present; positive capillary refill.
- **HEENT**
  - **Head/face:** Normocephalic; no lesions, tenderness, or masses; facial features symmetrical; no TMJ tenderness, locking, or clicking.
- **Eyes**
  - **Snellen:** R 20/25, L 20/20, both 20/20.
  - Extraocular muscles intact, no nystagmus.
  - Corneal light reflex symmetrical bilaterally.
  - Visual fields normal by confrontation.
  - Cornea and iris intact, anterior chamber clear.
  - Sclera white, conjunctivae clear and glossy.
  - Pupils equal, round, reactive to light and accommodation (PERRLA) direct and consensual.
  - Positive constriction and convergence.
  - Red reflex present bilaterally, discs flat with sharp margins, vessels present without crossing defects, retina even color without hemorrhages or exudates, macula even-colored.
- **Ears**
  - External ear skin intact; no masses, lesions, or discharge.
  - No tragus tenderness present.
  - Weber test: No lateralization.
  - Rinne test: Air conduction (AC) < bone conduction (BC).
  - Whisper test normal.
  - External ear canals clear without redness, swelling, lesions, or discharge.
  - Tympanic membranes intact, pearly gray with light reflex and landmarks visible.
- **Nose**
  - Nares patent, no sinus tenderness present.
  - Nasal mucosa pink.
  - Septum intact, no deviation.
- **Mouth**
  - Lips, oral mucosa, and gingivae pink and moist without lesions.
  - Teeth all present, clean, dental work present, no obvious caries.
  - Pharynx pink, tonsils +1, palate intact.
  - Tongue smooth, pink, symmetrical, no lesions.
- **Neck and axillae**
  - Thyroid not palpable.
  - Carotid pulses +2 and equal. No bruits, no jugular venous distension.
  - No lymphadenopathy of neck, axillae, or epitrochlear nodes.
  - Trachea midline, no abnormal masses or pulsations.
- **Thorax**
  - S_1; S_2; no S_3, S_4, murmurs, gallops, or thrills present.
  - PMI 1.5 cm at fifth intercostal space (ICS) at midclavicular line.
  - Anteroposterior less than transverse diameter, respiration unlabored.
  - Chest expansion symmetrical; no tenderness, scars, masses, or lesions.
  - Resonant percussion sound over lung fields.
  - Lungs clear, no adventitious breath sounds heard.
  - Breasts symmetrical; no masses, nipple discharge, or lymphadenopathy.
  - Normal spinal curvatures with no tenderness.
  - No costovertebral angle tenderness present.
- **Abdomen**
  - Abdomen slightly rounded, positive respiratory movement, no masses or pulsations observed.
  - Scar from previous surgery on right lower abdomen.
  - Bowel sounds present, no vascular sounds heard.

- Tympany in all four quadrants.
- Abdomen soft, no hepatomegaly, liver 10 cm at the midclavicular line, no splenomegaly, no masses or tenderness.
- No palpable lymph nodes in inguinal area.

- **Aorta 2 cm**
  - No femoral bruits; pulses 2+ and equal.
- **Musculoskeletal system and extremities**
  - Joints and muscles symmetrical.
  - Muscles well developed, +5 strength of upper and lower extremities.
  - Full ROM of upper and lower extremities.
  - Pulses 2+ bilaterally.
  - DTRs 2+; positive plantar reflex.
  - Skin warm, hair on both lower legs; no varicose veins; superficial and deep sensations intact.
  - Gait normal, heel-and-toe walk and deep knee bend without difficulty, negative Romberg.
- **Genitalia**
  - Circumcised male.
  - External genitalia without discharge, lesions, or abnormalities.
  - No scrotal swelling.
  - Testes smooth without masses.
  - No hernia present.
- **Rectum**
  - Perianal area intact without hemorrhoids.
  - Prostate smooth, firm, without masses +1.
  - Rectal wall smooth without masses or tenderness.
  - Stool brown and occult blood negative.

Significant findings that influence your plan of care:

- A 32-year-old white man who appears in no distress and in good health.
- Physical findings all normal.
- Smokes five to eight cigarettes a day; drinks beer in moderation.
- Diet is high in fat and cholesterol.
- Father died of sudden cardiac death at age 69 and had HTN.
- Is unaware of his BP or cholesterol level.
- Is exposed to environmental risks on the job, causing him to suffer three injuries in the last 5 years that needed treatment.
- Discusses problems with wife, but also states, "I try not to think about my problems."

3. List the positive and negative influences on Mr. Holsvick's health status at this time.

____

____

4. Cluster the supporting data for the following nursing diagnoses:

   a. Knowledge deficit related to health promotion activities.

   ____

   b. Risk of injury related to high-risk work environment.

   ____

5. Identify any additional nursing diagnoses for this patient.

____

____

6. Name a collaborative nursing diagnosis for this patient. Be specific about what the expected outcome of the diagnosis would include.

____

____

Chapter 23

Assessing the Mother-to-Be

Name ______________________ Date ______________

Course ______________________ Instructor ______________________

1. Many changes occur during pregnancy as a result of hormone changes and fetal growth. Match the changes in the first column with the appropriate definitions in the second column.

Changes	Definition
1. Chloasma	a. Increased salivation
2. Linea nigra	b. Nosebleeds
3. Striae gravidarum	c. Softening of cervix
4. Angioma	d. Craving unusual foods
5. Palmar erythema	e. Mask of pregnancy
6. Hirsutism	f. Heartburn
7. Epistaxis	g. Increased pigmentation of linea alba
8. Epulis	h. Increased hair growth
9. Ptyalism	i. Bluish discoloration of cervix
10. Pica	j. Separation of abdominal recti muscles
11. Pyrosis	k. Vascular spiders
12. Goodell's sign	l. Stretch marks
13. Chadwick's sign	m. Redness on palms of hands
14. Hegar's sign	n. Raised, red nodules on gums
15. Diastasis recti abdominis	o. Softening of uterus

2. Identify the following signs and symptoms as presumptive, probable, or positive of pregnancy.

   a. Fetal heart sounds ______________________

   b. Nausea ______________________

   c. Abdominal enlargement ______________________

   d. Breast tenderness ______________________

e. Hegar's sign ______

f. Chadwick's sign ______

g. Skin changes ______

h. Fatigue ______

i. Positive pregnancy test ______

j. Braxton-Hicks contractions ______

k. Visualization of fetus by ultrasound ______

l. Ballottement ______

m. Frequent urination ______

n. Quickening ______

o. Amenorrhea ______

3. You are taking your patient's health history. Name at least three diseases that are a cause for concern during pregnancy.

______

4. What additional assessments do you need to include in the prenatal assessment to monitor fetal development?

______

5. Your patient's last menstrual period (LMP) was 10/1/06. Calculate the estimated date of confinement using Naegele's rule (LMP + 7 days – 3 months).

______

6. What should you include in the postpartum assessment?

______

______

7. When assessing a pregnant patient, what changes or common findings might you see from head to toe?

______

______

8. Consider your own ethnic background. What, if any, cultural practices are associated with pregnancy and delivery?

______

______

Name ______________________ Date ____________

Course ______________________ Instructor ______________________

Abnormal Case Study: Sara Silverstone

Sara Silverstone, age 28, is a married elementary school teacher, gravida 1, para 1. She delivered a 9-lb boy by cesarean section owing to failure to progress. Spinal duramorph anesthesia was administered. She is admitted to the maternity unit with an intravenous line of 5 percent dextrose in lactated Ringer's solution 125 mL/hr infusing in her left hand. Because her condition is unstable, you perform a focused assessment.

Physical Assessment

- *General health status:* Temperature 99°F; awake, alert, oriented x 3; feels "wiped out" but happy.
- *Integumentary:* Skin color pale, nailbeds pale, capillary refill > 3 seconds, mucous membranes dry and pale, skin cool and clammy.
- *Respiratory:* Respirations 12/min and shallow.
- *Cardiovascular:* Tachycardia 118 beats per minute (BPM) and regular, blood pressure (BP) 90/50 mm Hg, positive systolic murmur 2/6, + 2 pulses.
- *Breasts:* Firm, increased venous pattern, dark areolae, nipples everted, plans to breastfeed.
- *Abdomen:* Distended, dressings dry and intact, no bowel sounds, abdomen tender, uterus soft at umbilicus, bleeding heavy with clots.
- *Genitourinary:* Foley catheter draining clear yellow urine.
- *Musculoskeletal:* Upper extremities +−5/5 muscle strength, lower extremities weak and numb.
- *Neurologic:* Lower extremities decreased sensation, "feel numb."

9. What assessment findings are cause for concern?

____

10. What assessment findings may signal a hemorrhage?

____

____

11. What assessment data are related to anesthesia and should be closely monitored?

____

12. What additional assessment data would be helpful in evaluating Mrs. Silverstone's fluid status?

____

13. Considering that this patient had a cesarean section, what additional system warrants close assessment?

____

14. When Mrs. Silverstone's condition stabilizes, what additional assessment data will be needed to plan her care?

____

____

15. Cluster the supporting data for the following nursing diagnoses:

    a. Fluid volume deficit related to bleeding.

    ____

    ____

    b. Risk for impaired ventilation.

    ____

    c. Risk for infection.

    ____

    d. Risk for pain.

    ____

16. List any additional nursing diagnoses.

____

____

Chapter 24

Assessing the Newborn and Infant

Name ______________________________ Date ______________

Course ______________________ Instructor ______________________

1. The newborn has many findings that are apparent at birth but disappear shortly after birth or within the first year of life. Match the findings in the first column with the appropriate definitions in the second column.

Findings	Definition
1. Acrocyanosis	a. Peeling of skin
2. Vernix caseosa	b. Small, white, pearl-like epithelial cysts on palate
3. Desquamation	c. White, cheesy substance on skin
4. Cutis marmorata	d. Dependent side of body red, nondependent side pale
5. Harlequin sign	e. Fine hair on face, back, and shoulders
6. Lanugo	f. Mottled skin
7. Milia	g. Hematoma between periosteum and skull
8. Epstein's pearls	h. Flat hemangioma at nape of neck
9. Craniosynostosis	i. Edema of soft scalp tissue from birth trauma
10. Stork bites	j. Premature closure of sutures
11. Caput succedaneum	k. Peripheral cyanosis
12. Cephalhematoma	l. White papules on face

2. What five areas are assessed with the Apgar score?

____

3. What areas do you need to include in the newborn's health history?

____

4. What measurements should you include in your assessment of the newborn and infant?

____

5. Match the reflexes in the first column to the proper techniques in the second column.

Reflex	**Technique**
1. Moro	a. Tap gently on forehead
2. Startle	b. Place your finger in infant's palm
3. Tonic neck	c. Stroke side of face
4. Palmar	d. Suddenly jar crib, or while holding infant in sitting position, let head drop back slightly
5. Plantar	e. Stroke lateral side of foot around to great toe
6. Babinski	f. Stroke lateral side of foot around to great toe
7. Stepping	g. Make a sudden loud noise
8. Crawling	h. With infant supine and leg extended, stimulate foot
9. Magnet	i. With infant prone, run fingers down sides of spine
10. Pull-to-sit	j. With leg flexed, apply pressure to sole of foot
11. Crossed extension	k. Place thumb against ball of foot
12. Trunk incurvation	l. With infant supine, turn head to one side
13. Rooting	m. Pull infant to sitting position
14. Sucking	n. Touch tip of infant's tongue
15. Extrusion	o. Touch infant's lip
16. Glabellar	p. Place infant on abdomen

6. When performing an assessment on a newborn or infant, what changes or common findings might you see from head to toe?

____

____

____

7. Consider your own ethnic background. What, if any, cultural practices are associated with care of the newborn?

____

____

Name ____________ Date ____________

Course ____________ Instructor ____________

Abnormal Case Study: Ryan Rogers

Martha Rogers, a 28-year-old, white, married woman, brings her 2-week-old son Ryan to the pediatrician's office. A full-term baby, Ryan had nursed well in the hospital, but now Mrs. Rogers is concerned. "Ryan's not keeping his feedings down," she states. "This is my first baby, and I'm afraid I must be doing something wrong." Ryan is lethargic and showing signs of dehydration. Considering the seriousness of his condition, you perform a focused assessment.

Health History

CHIEF COMPLAINT:

"Ryan's not keeping his feedings down."

Symptom Analysis:

P—Vomits within an hour after feeding.

Q—"Vomits across the room." Vomit is stale milk.

R—After he vomits, he wants to nurse again as if he is hungry. He seems to be getting more lethargic.

S—At first, he vomited every now and then, but now he seems to vomit after every feeding.

T—Vomiting started when he was 1 week old.

Past Health History:

- Pregnancy, labor, and delivery essentially uneventful.
- Apgar scores at birth 9/10, weight 8 lb.
- Began nursing right after delivery without problem.

Family History:

- Father had pyloric stenosis when he was 5 weeks old.

8. What factors in Ryan's history place him at risk for pyloric stenosis? Why?

____

____

____

9. Because the risk for dehydration is a concern, what additional questions should you ask Mrs. Rogers that would give clues to Ryan's hydration status?

____

____

____

Physical Assessment

- *General appearance:* Lethargic.
- *Vital signs:* Temperature 100°F, pulse 180 beats per minure (BPM), respirations 45/min, weight 7 lb.
- *Integumentary:* Poor turgor, skin warm and dry.
- *Head, eyes, ears, nose, and throat (HEENT):* Sunken fontanels, mucous membranes pink, but dry.
- *Respiratory:* Tachypnea, lungs clear.
- *Cardiovascular:* Tachycardia.
- *Abdomen:* Distended upper abdomen, visible reverse peristaltic waves in epigastric area, positive bowel sounds, palpable, olive-shaped mass in epigastric region.
- *Neurologic/musculoskeletal:* Weak, responds to tactile stimuli, not very active.

10. Which assessment findings suggest pyloric stenosis?

____

____

11. Which assessment findings suggest dehydration?

____

____

12. Considering Ryan's age, what developmental tasks (Erikson) would be appropriate at this stage?

____

13. Name one nursing intervention that would help Ryan maintain trust.

____

14. Cluster the supporting data for the following nursing diagnoses:

    a. Fluid volume deficit related to vomiting.

    ____

    ____

    b. Altered nutrition less than body requirements related to inability to retain feedings.

    ____

15. The following diagnosis is potential or at risk for. State a possible reason for this diagnosis: Risk for aspiration.

____

16. Identify any additional nursing diagnoses for Ryan.

____

____

Chapter 25

Assessing the Toddler and Preschooler

Name ______________________ Date ____________

Course ____________________ Instructor ______________________

1. The developmental task for the toddler is autonomy versus shame and doubt. What type of behaviors might you see if your patient has been successful at this stage? What type of behaviors might you see if she or he has been unsuccessful at this stage?

2. The developmental task for the preschooler is initiative versus guilt. What type of behaviors might you see if your patient has been successful at this stage? What type of behaviors might you see if he or she has been unsuccessful at this stage?

3. What are the major health issues for the toddler and preschooler?

4. Name six assessment findings that might lead you to suspect child abuse.

5. What factors should you consider when performing a physical assessment on a toddler or preschooler?

6. How does the physical exam differ from an adult's examination?

7. When performing an assessment on a toddler or preschooler, what changes or common findings might you see from head to toe?

____

____

8. Consider your own ethnic background. What are your culture's expectations for children?

____

Name ______________________ Date ______________

Course ______________ Instructor ______________________

Abnormal Case Study: Max Ingram

Max Ingram, age 15 months, is brought into the ED by his 17-year-old mother. She voices concern that he has a "high fever" and is chronically fussy and irritable. His admitting vital signs are as follows: temperature 101.2°F rectally, pulse 158 beats per minute (BPM), respirations 32/min, and blood pressure (BP) 112/74 mm Hg. Max weighs 20 lb and is 29.5 inches tall. He whines and clings to his mother throughout the history and physical exam, while she tries to get him to take a bottle of milk. You notice that besides his small size, his complexion is pale.

Health History

BIOGRAPHICAL DATA:

- 15-month-old white boy with one younger sibling.
- Health insurance: Medical card.
- Lives with single mother (17 years old, unemployed). Mother and children are living with a "good friend" at present until mother can find employment (friend's address provided and verified).

Current Health Status:

- Mother describes child's health as "okay" until past few months, when child developed increased fussiness, decreased activity tolerance, and trouble sleeping.
- Mother reports increased respiratory infections and claims child "feels feverish a lot." Is unable to be specific regarding circumstances (does not have thermometer).

Past Health History:

- No prenatal care until third trimester; forceps delivery with epidural after 18-hour labor.
- Infant born "a few weeks early" but went home with mother at discharge; unsure of Apgar score; reports infant cried at birth and fed without difficulty.
- Hospitalized for respiratory syncytial virus at 6 months; treated for three episodes of otitis media in first year (unsure of dates/age of infant at time). Claims he has "lots of colds."
- Has not had immunizations beyond his "second set after he was born."
- No medications other than antibiotics; gives Tylenol if "feverish" or fussy; has given "purple" over-the-counter (OTC) cold medication (unsure of name).
- Denies known allergies to medications, but thinks child has allergies or asthma.

Family History:

- Mother describes her health as "good." Says she "gets colds once or twice a year."
- Maternal grandfather left family when mother was 8 years old; health unknown.
- Maternal grandmother's health "poor" secondary to arthritis and "mental problems."
- Mother reports her three older siblings are in "good" health.
- Child's father's health "good" as far as is known. Mother does not maintain contact with him (same father for both children).
- Paternal grandfather died in auto accident in his 30s—no known health problems.
- Paternal grandmother is in her 60s and has diabetes mellitus.
- Multiple paternal siblings—health unknown.

Review of Systems:

- *General health status:* More fussy and irritable than usual, more colds than usual, sleeping poorly.
- *Integumentary:* Denies changes in skin, hair, or nails.

- *Head, eyes, ears, nose, and throat (HEENT):* Tugs at ears; denies hoarseness, rubbing eyes, or excessive tearing/redness.
- *Respiratory:* More frequent colds.
- *Cardiovascular:* Can feel "heart racing and pounding in his chest," especially with crying/exertion.
- *Gastrointestinal:* Occasional diarrhea/vomiting that never lasts beyond 1 day.
- *Genitourinary:* Circumcised, urinates without difficulty.
- *Musculoskeletal:* Denies difficulties/concerns.
- *Neurologic:* Denies seizure-like activity, feels child hears and sees okay.
- *Lymphatic:* More frequent episodes of colds; worries it's because he's behind on shots.

Psychosocial Profile:

- *Self-care activities:* Holds own bottle, feeds self, indicates wants by pointing/fussing.
- *Nutritional patterns:* Switched to "regular milk" (unsure if whole) at about 10 to 11 months for convenience and because less expensive. Child still drinks from bottle—about eight 8-oz bottles per day. "Picky eater but loves milk." Occasionally eats toast, applesauce, cereal. Seldom offers water because child usually refuses. Mother not concerned about weight because she was "tiny" as a child. *24-hour dietary recall:* Breakfast—8 oz milk, $\frac{1}{4}$ cup applesauce. Midmorning—>8 oz milk. Lunch—$\frac{1}{4}$ cup Ramen noodles without broth, >8 oz milk. Afternoon—8-oz milk bottle for nap, 8 oz Pepsi on awakening. Supper—Refused pizza, >8 oz milk, cookie. Bedtime—8 oz milk for bedtime. Mother claims this is fairly typical, usually eats a little more but appetite has diminished. Occasionally wants bottle if awakens at night.
- *Activity/exercise patterns:* Says he is not an active child. Prefers to play quietly and spends most time indoors watching TV. Describes him as quiet and slow to warm up to people but generally a "good baby."
- *Elimination:* Still in diapers, has semisolid light brown bowel movement daily or less, denies constipation, has occasional diarrhea/vomiting.
- *Sleep/rest patterns:* Sleeps about 8 to 10 hours per night with two or three daytime naps lasting 1 to 3 hours. Gives bottle to help sleep; puts child to bed about 9 P.M. (denies routine), and child spontaneously awakens about 7 or 8 A.M. and plays quietly until mother gets him up around 9 A.M. Usually sleeps "okay" with occasional awakening but self-soothes back to sleep; more fussy past few months when awakening at night.
- *Personal habits:* Starting to put things in mouth, including dirt and small debris he finds on floor. Mother smokes about 10 to 20 cigarettes a day. Child permitted to have soft drinks—limits to one bottle of soda per day because she feels more would not be good for him.
- *Occupational health patterns:* Child is dependent on mother for needs. Mother applied for assistance about 3 months ago but has not followed up. Mother did not finish high school; claims she wants to find a job, but unless she can find affordable and accessible child care, she is limited in what she does and where she works.
- *Environmental health patterns:* Family lives in "very old house" with peeling paint and loose plaster, but mother denies noticing if child ingests any. Has tried to ensure that cleaning supplies and medications are kept out of child's reach. Stairways are open, but child "ignores them" or stays away if she yells at him. Lives on busy street, so child usually is kept inside, although there is a small, fenced backyard where child occasionally plays. Friend's car is equipped with seatbelts, which they don't use, and children do not have car safety seats.
- *Roles/relationships:* Mother claims to have loving relationship with child. Child described as a "good baby" who does not give her "much grief." Child's father never lived with family and has no contact. Family currently lives with male friend of mother's. Mother claims he gets along with her children "okay" and denies abuse/violence. No contact with maternal relatives except child's aunt (mother's older sister), who sometimes helps them with money and clothes.
- *Stress and coping:* Child cries/fusses when uncomfortable or upset. Mother soothes him with a bottle or will give Tylenol (assumes he feels bad); disciplines by smacking hands or telling "no." Child is usually compliant and seldom has to be spanked/scolded.

9. What information from the health history indicates that Max is at risk for a nutritional deficiency?

____

10. What information from the 24-hour dietary recall indicates a nutritional deficiency?

____

11. What factors from Max's history increase his risk for an ear infection?

____

____

12. Aside from the nutritional deficit, what other health problems is Max at risk for?

____

Physical Assessment

- *General appearance:* Generally passive/withdrawn; whimpers and clings to mother with no vigorous objection to health-care providers; pale, sits limply in mother's lap; appears small for age.
- *Vital signs:* Temperature 101.2°F (rectal); pulse 158 BPM; respirations 32/min; full/deep; BP 112/74 mm Hg; weight 20 lb, height 29.5 inches.
- *Integumentary:* Skin warm and moist; nails spoon-shaped, brittle.
- *HEENT:*
  - Normocephalic with fine, evenly distributed hair; scalp dry/flaky.
  - Pupils equal, responsive to light; light reflexes equal; follows object through all fields; sclerae white, conjunctivae pale.
  - Dirty behind ears; scant light brown cerumen bilaterally; tympanic membranes bulging and red with little mobility.
  - Nose aligned midline, no septal deviation, membranes pale/moist.
  - Dentition present and showing signs of decay consistent with prolonged bottle feeding; tongue midline, gag intact; throat pink, without exudate/erythema.
  - Mild lymphadenopathy.
- *Respiratory:* Rate 32/min and labored, breath sounds equal bilaterally, clear to auscultation; mild grunting.
- *Cardiovascular:* Marked precordial pulsation; point of maximal impulse readily visible and palpable lateral to midclavicular line in sixth intercostal space (ICS); rate 158 BPM, regular.
- *Gastrointestinal:* Bowel sounds present, regular, although slightly diminished; no signs of distress with palpation; no palpable masses.
- *Genitourinary:* Normal male genitalia; meatus midline and nonerythematous, testes descended bilaterally; anus normal.
- *Musculoskeletal:* Minimal muscle resistance; full passive range of motion (ROM); extremities symmetrical, no joint swelling/inflammation; stands and walks to return to mother; gait normal for age.
- *Neurologic:* Cranial nerves intact; deep tendon reflexes (DTRs) equal/diminished; developmentally delayed.

13. What assessment findings suggest that Max may have another ear infection?

____

14. What assessment findings suggest that Max may have anemia?

____

15. Max's mother says she can feel his heart racing and pounding in his chest. What might account for the marked precordial pulsation and rapid heart rate?

____

16. Identify teaching needs for Max's mother.

____

17. Considering Max's age, what developmental tasks (Erikson) would be appropriate at this stage?

____

18. Name one developmental task for this developmental stage.

____

19. Cluster the supporting data for the following nursing diagnosis:

   a. Altered nutrition less than body requirements related to poor dietary intake.

   ____

20. The following diagnoses are potential or at risk for. State a possible reason for each diagnosis:

   a. Potential complication: hyperthermia related to infection.

   ____

   b. Risk for infection related to increased susceptibility.

   ____

   c. Risk for injury.

   ____

21. Identify any additional nursing diagnoses for Max.

____

____

Chapter 26

Assessing the School-Age Child and Adolescent

Name ____________		Date ____________	
Course ____________	Instructor ____________		

1. The developmental task for the school-age child is industry versus inferiority. What type of behavior might you see if your patient has been successful at this stage? What type of behavior might you see if she or he has been unsuccessful at this stage?

____

____

2. The developmental task for the adolescent is identity versus role diffusion. What type of behavior might you see if your patient has been successful at this stage? What type of behavior might you see if he or she has been unsuccessful at this stage?

____

____

3. What health concerns should you screen for during your assessment?

____

4. Identify areas of health teaching for school-age and adolescent patients.

____

5. How does the physical exam differ from an adult's?

____

____

6. When assessing a school-age child or adolescent, what changes or common findings might you see from head to toe?

____

____

7. Consider your ethnic background. What is your culture's expectation for adolescents?

____

Name ______________________ Date ____________

Course ____________________ Instructor ____________________

Abnormal Case Study: Nathan Lyons

Nathan Lyons, age 10, is admitted to the hospital with acute lymphocytic leukemia. His mother states that he was fine until a few weeks ago, when he began complaining that he was tired all the time. He also noticed that his gums bled when he brushed his teeth and that he had bruises on his arms but couldn't remember hurting them.

Health History

CHIEF COMPLAINT:

"I'm tired all the time."

Symptom Analysis:

P—No precipitating event, some relief with rest.

Q—"Just tired, no energy."

R—Related signs/symptoms include bleeding gums and bruising.

S—Seems to be getting worse.

T—Started a few weeks ago.

Past Health History:

- Frequent ear infections until age 6.
- No surgeries, hospitalizations, or trauma.
- Immunizations up-to-date.
- Allergies: No known drug allergies; has had penicillin without reaction, no food or environmental allergies.
- No medications.

Family History:

- Family history of leukemia.

Review of Systems:

- *General health status:* Fatigue, loss of appetite, weight loss of a couple of pounds in the past month.
- *Integumentary:* Unexplained bruising.
- *Head, eyes, ears, nose, and throat (HEENT):* Bleeding gums, "lumps" in neck.
- *Respiratory:* Shortness of breath with activity.
- *Cardiovascular:* No complaints.
- *Musculoskeletal:* Weakness.
- *Neurologic:* No complaints.

Psychosocial Profile:

- *Health patterns/beliefs:* Always has annual check-up. Mother says, "I always try to be proactive."
- *Typical day:* Awakens at 7 A.M., has breakfast, leaves for school by 8 A.M. Has classes until 3 P.M.; participates in after-school sports until 5 P.M. Dinner at 6 P.M., homework 7 to 9 P.M.; then takes shower and goes to bed by 10 P.M. Does well in school.
- *Nutritional patterns: 24-hour recall:* Breakfast—4 oz orange juice, cereal with milk. Lunch—Peanut butter and jelly sandwich, cookies, milk. Snack—Fruit snack and milk. Dinner—Hamburger, French fries, chocolate cake.
- *Sleep/rest patterns:* Sleeps 9 hours uninterrupted.
- *Activity/exercise patterns:* Loves sports, uses protective equipment.
- *Environmental health patterns:* Home environment has safety alarms and smoke detectors; lives in suburbs.
- *Religious/cultural influences:* Protestant; English heritage, no cultural influence on health.
- *Social supports:* Family, school friends.

Physical Assessment

- *General appearance:* Awake, alert, oriented x 3, color pale, looks tired.

- *Vital signs:* Temperature 99°F, pulse 104 beats per minute (BPM), respirations 22/min, blood pressure (BP) 100/60 mm Hg.
- *Integumentary:* Skin color pale, mucous membranes and conjunctiva pale, several bruises (3 cm) noted on arms bilaterally, no other lesions.
- *HEENT:* Gums bleeding, positive cervical lymphadenopathy.
- *Respiratory:* Lungs clear.
- *Cardiovascular:* heart regular rate and rhythm, tachycardia, systolic murmur II/VI.
- *Abdomen*: Positive splenomegaly and hepatomegaly.
- *Musculoskeletal/neurologic:* Able to move all extremities, but generalized weakness.

8. Identify the assessment data that may indicate anemia or bleeding.

 ____

 ____

9. Identify the assessment data that may indicate infection.

 ____

10. Considering anemia, bleeding, and infection are common complications of acute lymphocytic leukemia, identify pertinent nursing diagnoses.

 ____

 ____

 ____

11. Cluster the supporting data for the following nursing diagnoses:

 a. Altered nutrition less than body requirements.

 ____

 b. Fatigue related to inadequate tissue perfusion secondary to anemia.

 ____

12. Identify any additional nursing diagnoses for Nathan.

 ____

13. Considering Nathan's age, what developmental tasks (Erikson) would be appropriate at this stage?

 ____

14. Identify a developmental task for this stage of development.

 ____

Name ______________________________ Date ______________

Course ______________________ Instructor ______________________

Abnormal Case Study: Sally Randolph

Sally Randolph, age 18, presents to your clinic complaining of amenorrhea for 7 months. Sally is a college freshman on a track athletic scholarship. She says she is usually healthy, has no other symptoms, and has not lost weight. She exercises daily by running 12 miles in the morning at 6:00 A.M. and 12 miles in the evening at 6:00 P.M., and she eats three meals a day. She comes from a large farm family, is the oldest of five children, and is the first in her family to go to college. She has been a track athlete for 2 years.

Health History

CHIEF COMPLAINT:

"I'm worried because I haven't had my period in 7 months, and I want to find out if something is wrong."

Current Health Status:

- No recent weight loss.
- Denies problems with appetite, has a healthy diet, denies anorexia or bulimia symptoms.
- Denies being sexually active.
- Before amenorrhea, her periods were light and lasted for about 5 days.

15. Considering Sally's history, what first comes to mind as a contributing factor to her amenorrhea?

____

Past Health History:

- Menarche age 16.
- Has never been sexually active and has never used oral contraceptives.
- Has never sustained any physical trauma.
- Has never had surgery.
- Was anemic, but it was 1 year ago.
- Only medication she takes is a multivitamin.
- Has never had a gynecological examination.
- No history of vaginal or reproductive organ infections.

Family History:

- Both parents alive and well.
- Three younger brothers and one younger sister, all healthy.

Psychosocial Profile:

- *Nutritional/weight patterns:* Good appetite, eats at least three meals a day, no recent weight gain or loss, fluid intake exceeds 2 L/day.
- *Activity/exercise patterns:* Runs 12 miles every morning and evening year round. Rarely does any other form of exercise.
- *Sleep/rest patterns:* Sleeps about 7 hours each night.
- *Personal habits:* Does not drink alcohol or use tobacco products.
- *Environmental health patterns:* Lives in college residence hall with one roommate; first time away from home for more than 1 week; comes from small farming community.

16. Considering the age of menarche for Sally, how else might you explain her amenorrhea?

____

17. Would this amenorrhea be considered primary or secondary?

____

Physical Assessment

- *General appearance:* Appears younger than 18 years; affect is appropriate; she is communicative and willing to undergo examination.
- *Height:* 5 feet, 1 inch.
- *Weight:* 100 lb.

Inspection:

- *Integumentary:* Hair distribution appropriate for maturational level.
- *Genitalia:* No lesions, other signs of infection, or obvious congenital abnormalities.
- Cervix is midline, clear, and pink and without lesions; os is patent.

Palpation:

- *Genitalia:* No swelling or induration of labia, urethral meatus, Skene's glands, or Bartholin's gland. Vaginal muscle tone strong.
- *Bimanual:* Cervix mobile, nontender; uterus small, pear-shaped, firm, mobile, nontender, anteverted.
- *Adnexa:* Ovaries firm bilaterally, mobile, and nontender.

18. Aside from amenorrhea, are there any other findings that warrant further investigation?

____

19. Considering Sally's age, what developmental tasks (Erikson) would be appropriate at this stage?

____

20. Identify a developmental task for this stage of development.

____

21. The following diagnoses are potential or at risk for. State the reasoning for each possible diagnosis:

    a. Risk for altered nutritional pattern less than bodily requirements.

    ____

    b. Risk for altered health maintenance related to inadequate understanding of exercise and menstrual cycle.

    ____

22. Identify any additional nursing diagnoses.

____

____

Chapter 27

Assessing the Older Adult

Name ______________________ Date ____________

Course ____________________ Instructor ____________________

1. Identify three factors that may confuse symptoms reported by older adults.

2. What might you do differently when obtaining a history from an older patient?

3. The developmental task for the older patient is integrity versus despair. What type of behavior might you see if your patient has been successful at this stage? What type of behavior might you see if she or he has been unsuccessful at this stage?

4. List five factors that you should consider when performing a physical assessment on an older patient.

5. When performing an assessment on an older patient, what changes might you see from head to toe?

6. Match the types of incontinence in the first column with the definitions in the second column.

Types of Incontinence	Definitions
1. Stress	a. Urine leakage resulting from inability to get to bathroom because of cognitive or physical impairment
2. Urge	b. Involuntary loss of urine with increased intra-abdominal pressure
3. Overflow	c. Leakage of urine resulting from inability to delay voiding
4. Functional	d. Leakage of urine from an overdistended bladder

7. Consider your ethnic background. What is your culture's view of the role of the older adult in the family and in society? How is the older adult cared for?

____

Name ______________________ Date ______________

Course ______________ Instructor ______________

Abnormal Case Study: Arthur O'Reilly

Arthur O'Reilly, age 65, has degenerative joint disease (DJD) and is being admitted to the orthopedic unit for total knee replacement. A retired floor installer and refinisher, the patient lives with his wife and has a 30-year-old son who lives nearby.

Health History

CHIEF COMPLAINT:

"The pain in my knee is getting worse, and I can hardly get around."

Symptom Analysis:

P—Pain with activity, pain is worse when the weather is bad, some relief with rest and medication.

Q—Dull, aching persistent pain.

R—Knees.

S—8/10, unrelenting.

T—Started 5 years ago.

Past Health History:

- Had measles, mumps, chickenpox, and rubella but unable to remember specifics.
- Inguinal hernia repair at age 45, torn medial collateral ligaments at age 50, no hospitalizations.
- History of hypertension (HTN).
- No known drug allergies; has had penicillin without reaction; no food or environmental allergies.
- Nonsteroidal anti-inflammatory drugs (celecoxib [Celebrex]) for arthritis; furosemide (Lasix), 20 mg once daily, for HTN.

Family History:

- Family history of HTN, cardiovascular disease, and DJD.

Review of Systems:

- *General health status:* Usually feels okay except when knee is hurting.
- *Integumentary:* No reported problems.
- *Head, eyes, ears, nose, and throat (HEENT):* No reported problems.
- *Respiratory:* No reported problems.
- *Cardiovascular:* No chest pain or palpitations; last electrocardiogram (ECG) 1 year ago was normal.
- *Genitourinary:* No reported problems.
- *Musculoskeletal:* Weakness in lower extremities, difficulty walking.
- *Neurologic:* No reported problems.

Psychosocial Profile:

- *Health patterns and beliefs/self-care activities:* Usually sees physician only when sick, but is seen every few months for HTN.
- *Typical day:* Awakens at 7 A.M., eats breakfast with wife, reads paper, works in garden until lunch, takes nap in afternoon, has dinner, watches TV until 11 P.M., and goes to bed.
- *Activity/exercise patterns:* Not as active as usual because of knee pain; has to use a cane.
- *Sleep/rest patterns:* Usually gets 7 to 8 hours of sleep a night, but awakens at times with knee pain.
- *Occupational health patterns:* Retired.
- *Roles, relationships, self-concept:* Married 32 years; says he feels like a "cripple."
- *Cultural/religious influences*: Irish Catholic; goes to church several times a week.
- *Sexuality patterns:* Knee pain sometimes affects sexual activity.
- *Social supports:* Wife and son are major sources of support. Has been married for 32 years.

Physical Assessment

- *General appearance:* Well-developed, obese man; appears stated age. Responds appropriately, affect pleasant. Ambulates with cane.
- *Vital signs:* Temperature 98.6°F, pulse 80 beats per minute (BPM), respirations 18/min, blood pressure (BP) 150/90 mm Hg, height 6 feet, weight 250 lb.
- *Integumentary:* Skin intact, warm, dry, and pink; several seborrhea keratosis lesions on upper torso.
- *HEENT:*
  - Head: Symmetrical midline.
  - Eyes: Vision 20/20 with corrective lenses, extraocular muscles intact, peripheral vision intact, funduscopic examination within normal limits.
  - Ears: Hearing intact, tympanic membrane intact and pearly gray, no drainage.
  - Nose: Patent, no drainage.
  - Mouth and throat: Mucous membranes pink, moist, and intact, no lesions; has upper partial bridge.
- *Respiratory:* Lungs clear.
- *Cardiovascular:* Regular rate and rhythm (heart regular rate and rhythm) $+S_4$, +2 pulses.
- *Abdomen:* Large and round, soft, nontender, positive bowel sounds, no organomegaly.
- *Musculoskeletal:* Full range of motion (ROM) of upper extremities, decreased ROM of knees, positive crepitus and swelling, +4/5 muscle strength lower extremities, +5/5 upper extremities.
- *Neurologic:* Awake, alert, oriented x 3, gait unsteady related to DJD, cranial nerves (CNs) I to XII intact, sensory intact, +2 deep tendon reflexes (DTRs).

8. Considering Mr. O'Reilly's age, what developmental tasks (Erikson) would be appropriate at this stage?

____

9. How might Mr. O'Reilly's illness affect his ability to be successful at this stage of development?

____

10. Mr. O'Reilly has DJD. How does this differ from rheumatoid arthritis?

____

11. From Mr. O'Reilly's history, identify risk factors for DJD.

____

12. From Mr. O'Reilly's physical assessment findings, identify signs of DJD.

____

____

13. Cluster the supporting data for the following nursing diagnoses.

    a. Pain related to physical activity.

    ____

    b. Impaired physical mobility related to pain and weakness.

    ____

    c. Sleep pattern disturbance related to pain.

    ____

14. Identify any additional nursing diagnoses for Mr. O'Reilly.

    ____

    ____

Answers

Some questions may have additional answers. Check the appropriate chapter in the text.

Chapter 1 Health Assessment and the Nurse

1. Nausea: Subjective
   Cyanosis: Objective
   Jaundice: Objective
   Edema: Objective
   Numbness: Subjective
   Diaphoresis: Objective
   Pallor: Objective
   Ptosis: Objective
   Dizziness: Subjective
   Stridor: Objective
   Palpitations: Subjective
   Irregular pulse: Objective
   Shortness of breath: Subjective
   Chest pain: Subjective

2. a. Lauren
   b. Mother, old records
   c. "My ear hurts" and irritable
   d. 2-year-old girl with 103°F temperature, cough, runny nose, decreased sleep and oral intake, tugging at ear, history of otitis media x 3

3. 1. c
   2. f
   3. g
   4. h
   5. b
   6. d
   7. a
   8. e

4. a. "What does it feel like, and when did it start? Point to where it hurts."
   b. "Would you like to talk about this?"
   c. "What makes you feel this way? Would you like to talk about it?"
   d. "What has your doctor said?"
   e. "I'm here now. How can I help you?"

5.

Communication Problem	**Correct Question/Statement**
a. Leading patient	"Can you point to where it hurts?"
b. Giving advice	"What do you feel is best?"
c. Offering false reassurance	"You seem concerned, would you like to talk about it?"
d. Using medical jargon	"You're going to have your ovaries removed through a laparoscope. The doctor will make a couple of small incisions..."
e. Using clichés	"Would you like to talk about this?"
f. Asking more than one question at a time	"What seems to be the problem?"

g. Taking responses personally	"I can see that you're upset. How can I help you?"
h. Changing the subject	"Would you like to talk about this?"
i. Assuming	Review the entire preoperative phase with your patient regardless of his or her educational level.
j. Feeling uncomfortable with subject	"Would you like to talk about this?"
k. Assuming rather than clarifying	"Was there a problem with taking your medications?"

6. a. Rose Montefalco.
   b. Old records.
   c. "My chest is killing me; it feels like I'm in a vice." Pain severity 10/10, down to 8/10 after nitroglycerin administration; difficulty breathing.
   d. Blood pressure (BP) 170/110 mm Hg; pulse 118 beats per minute (BPM), regular; respirations 32/min; temperature 99.8°F; pulse oximetry 90 percent on room air; cardiac monitor shows sinus tachycardia with occasional premature ventricular contractions. BP 160/100 mm Hg; pulse 110 BPM; respirations 28/min; pulse oximetry 93 percent on 3 L of oxygen after nitroglycerin.

7. S—"My chest is killing me; it feels like I'm in a vice."
   O—78-year-old woman; BP 170/110 mm Hg; pulse 118 BPM, regular; respirations 32/min; temperature 99.8°F; pulse oximetry 90 percent on room air. Monitor shows sinus tachycardia with occasional premature ventricular contractions. Diaphoretic, pale, and clammy.
   A—Chest pain, altered cardiovascular status, and ineffective breathing.
   P—Relieve pain, establish effective breathing, and stabilize cardiovascular status.
   I—Continue to monitor, obtain diagnostic test results, titrate nitroglycerin, continue oxygen.
   E—Vital signs more stable, pulse oximetry 93 percent on 3 L of oxygen, chest pain 8/10.

8. D—"My chest is killing me..."; 78-year-old woman; BP 170/110 mm Hg; pulse 118 BPM, regular; respirations 32/min; temperature 99.8°F; pulse oximetry 90 percent on room air. Monitor shows sinus tachycardia with occasional premature ventricular contractions. Diaphoretic, pale, and clammy.
   A—Oxygen at 3 L, cardiac monitor, intravenous nitroglycerin, obtain diagnostic tests.
   R—Chest pain 8/10 after start of nitroglycerin; BP 160/100 mm Hg; pulse 110 BPM; respirations 28/min; pulse oximetry 93 percent on 3 L of oxygen.

9. P—Chest pain, ineffective breathing, altered cardiovascular status.
   I—Oxygen at 3 L; intravenous nitroglycerin; continue cardiac monitoring; obtain diagnostic tests.
   E—Chest pain 8/10 after intravenous nitroglycerin; BP 160/100 mm Hg; pulse 110 BPM; respirations 28/min; pulse oximetry 93 percent on 3 L of oxygen.

10. Not specific

11. 1
    1
    3
    3
    2

Chapter 2 The Health History

1. a. Biographical data
   b. Biographical data
   c. Family history
   d. Current health status
   e. Biographical data
   f. Psychosocial profile
   g. Past health history
   h. Psychosocial profile
   i. Review of systems
   j. Past health history
   k. Review of systems
   l. Past health history
   m. Current health status
   n. Psychosocial profile
   o. Review of systems
   p. Biographical data
   q. Review of systems
   r. Biographical data
   s. Psychosocial profile
   t. Review of systems
   u. Psychosocial profile
   v. Review of systems
   w. Biographical data
   x. Psychosocial profile
   y. Review of systems

2. 1. e
   2. a
   3. b
   4. c
   5. g
   6. h
   7. f
   8. d

Chapter 3 Approach to the Physical Assessment

1. 1. d
   2. e
   3. a
   4. b
   5. c
   6. k
   7. j
   8. l
   9. f
   10. h
   11. i
   12. g

2. a. Bimanual palpation
   b. Palpation
   c. Percussion
   d. Inspection
   e. Auscultation
   f. Palpation
   g. Ballottement
   h. Ballottement
   i. Fist percussion
   j. Percussion
   k. Auscultation
   l. Palpation

3. a. Balls or ulnar surface
   b. Dorsal part
   c. Finger pads/tips

4. The difference in weight and subsequent thickness of the chest wall may account for the difference in breath sounds, although both are normal. When assessing for abnormalities, use the patient as her or his own comparative.

5. Infants: Have parent hold infant; do otoscopic and funduscopic exams last.
   Preschoolers: Have parent present; use toys, games, or demonstrate on dolls.
   Adolescents: Ask if they want parent present (may be modest and say no).
   Pregnant patients: Assess mother and fetus; include fundal height and fetal heart tone.
   Older adults: Avoid certain exam positions if patient has trouble assuming them; allow for vision and hearing deficits.

6. a. Lithotomy or dorsal recumbent
   b. Flexed at hips leaning over table
   c. Supine
   d. Standing
   e. Sitting
   f. Supine or sitting
   g. Sims' or flexed at hips leaning over

7. a. High
   b. High
   c. Low
   d. Low
   e. High

8. Cast or injury to arm, intravenous access, side of mastectomy, vascular access

9. All systems are related, so they can affect or be affected by every system. If a problem occurs in one system, you may see changes in other systems, or vice versa.

Chapter 4 Assessing Pain

1. a. Myth
   b. Truth
   c. Myth
   d. Myth
   e. Truth
   f. Myth

2. a. Mechanical
   b. Thermal
   c. Chemical

d. Mechanical
e. Mechanical
f. Thermal

3. 1. b
2. c
3. e
4. a
5. d

4. 1. c
2. a
3. d
4. b

5. P—What were you doing before the headache started? Did anything make the headache better or worse?
Q—What does it feel like?
R—Can you show me where it hurts?
S—On a scale of 0 to 10, how bad is the pain?
T—When did it start? How long does it last? Have you ever done this before?

6. a. CRIES scale
b. FACES pain scale
c. Numeric scale 0 to 10
d. PAINAD

Chapter 5 Approach to the Mental Health Assessment

1. a. Dementia
b. Delirium or depression
c. Depression
d. Dementia
e. Dementia

2. 1. Lives alone
2. Poor health
3. Limited finances
4. Drug or alcohol abuse
5. Social isolation

3. 1. Poor eye contact
2. Slumped posture
3. Poor grooming

4. 1. Feelings of hopelessness: How have you been feeling? What are your plans for tomorrow?
2. Suicidal ideations: Have you ever thought about hurting yourself?
3. Plan for suicide: If the patient has suicidal ideations, does she have a plan?
4. Possessions: Has the patient been putting affairs in order? Giving things away?
5. Auditory hallucinations: Are you hearing voices that tell you to hurt yourself?
6. Lack of support network: Is the patient isolated?
7. Alcohol or substance abuse: Is the patient drinking or taking drugs?
8. Precipitating event: Has the patient experienced a recent loss?

5. 1. Perception of the event: How are you feeling? How have you been since your husband passed?
   2. Supports: Do you have family? Friends? Church? Community?
   3. Coping mechanims: What have you been doing to manage? Can you talk about how you are feeling?

6. 1. History of mood disorder
   2. Low self-esteem
   3. Unwanted pregnancy
   4. Unemployment
   5. Poor marital relationship
   6. Depressed father
   7. Poor supports
   8. External stressors

7. Marks on neck, complaints of headaches, red eyes, belts, locked doors, or disorientation after being alone

8. 1. d
   2. i
   3. h
   4. e
   5. j
   6. a
   7. b
   8. c
   9. f
   10. g

9. C—Have you ever felt you should cut down on your drinking?
   A—Have people annoyed you by criticizing your drinking?
   G—Have you ever felt guilty about your drinking?
   E—Have you ever had an eye opener?

Chapter 6 Teaching the Patient

1. Educational level, financial resources, and current health status (e.g., pain, age, stress, and available supports)

2. Vision, hearing, cognitive ability, motor skills, breathing problems, and muscle strength

3. Obesity, hypertension (HTN), non–insulin-dependent diabetes mellitus (NIDDM), diet, noncompliance with taking prescribed medications

4. Independent, has full-time job with medical insurance coverage, has supportive family

5. a. BP 180/100 mm Hg; glucose 160 mg/dL; overweight with poor diet; urinary signs and symptoms; missed medications; inconsistent glucose monitoring; jokes during exam; thinks she has a urinary tract infection and needs antibiotic so she can get back to work.

   b. Missed medications; inconsistent glucose monitoring; overweight with poor diet; jokes during exam; thinks she has a urinary tract infection and needs antibiotic so she can get back to work.

6. The plan has to fit in with her work schedule.

Chapter 7 Assessing Wellness

1. Supports: Family, friends, organized groups.
   Psychological state: Patient needs not only the information but also to believe that it is important. Depression, anxiety, or stress may also affect health behaviors.
2. Barriers to health-care: Lack of money; lack of transportation; distant location of health-care; and ethnic, gender, or age discrimination
3. Exercising right before bedtime may make it difficult to fall asleep.
   Nicotine increases the time needed to fall asleep and causes lighter sleep.
   Caffeine increases sleep latency and decreases total sleep time.
   Alcohol affects the rapid-eye-movement sleep cycle and fragments sleep.
   Obesity increases the risk for sleep apnea. Gaining weight increases sleep, and losing weight decreases sleep.
   High-protein foods increase alertness; high-carbohydrate foods increase relaxation.
   Stress decreases the ability to sleep.
   Congestive heart failure can cause nocturnal dyspnea; pain associated with surgery can interrupt sleep.
4. 1. c
   2. a
   3. e
   4. f
   5. b
   6. d
5. Maximum = 145; minimum = 87; ideal = 116
6. Infant: Unmet basic needs
   Toddler: Separation from parents (e.g., owing to hospitalization)
   School-age child: School
   Adolescent: Physical changes of puberty; sexuality
   Young adult: Relationships and work
   Middle-aged adult: Family and finances
   Older adult: Retirement, illness, and finances
7. Infant: Choking, accidental poisoning
   Preschool/school-age child: Accidents related to bikes, sports
   Adolescent: Accidents related to driving; health problems related to drugs or sex
   Young adult/middle-aged adult: Work-related injuries
   Older adult: Falls

Chapter 8 Assessing Nutrition

1. 1. c
   2. a
   3. e
   4. b
   5. d
   6. g
   7. f
2. Excess water-soluble vitamins are excreted from the body. Fat-soluble vitamins are not excreted, so they can build up to toxic levels.

3. Vitamin A: Fat-soluble
   Vitamin B: Water-soluble
   Vitamin C: Water-soluble
   Vitamin D: Fat-soluble
   Vitamin E: Fat-soluble
   Vitamin K: Fat-soluble

4. Infant/toddler: Fats for nervous system development
   Preschool child: Iron to prevent iron-deficiency anemia (common in this age group)
   School-age child: Calcium for prepubertal bone development
   Adolescent: Iron for girls to prevent anemia resulting from menstruation; calcium for bone development
   Pregnant woman: Increased calories, milk, fluids, and vitamins (especially iron and folic acid) for fetal development
   Older adult: Calcium to decrease risk for osteoporosis, especially in postmenopausal women; decreased calories to prevent obesity, an increased risk in this age group

7. Cancer is always a possibility when an older patient presents with unexplained weight loss. Because weight loss is a symptom of prostate cancer, rule this out first. Mr. Liang does not describe symptoms consistent with prostate concerns of any type, however. He himself has provided an important perspective on his weight loss—he says he doesn't like American food.

8. Diet lacking in fruits, vegetables, dairy, and meats with an overabundance of grains; should consider whole grains; deficit in fluid intake

9. Inadequate diet and dehydration

10. Digital rectal examination of the prostate and prostate-specific antigen test.

11. Urinary complaints; enlarged, irregular, hard prostate; possible changes in bowel habits; possible back pain; and positive inguinal nodes if metastatic

12. Fatigue, diet and loss of appetite, low BP, increased pulse and respirations, pale conjunctiva, positive systolic murmur 2/6, and low hematocrit and hemoglobin

13. Approximate percent weight loss is 17 percent; approximate body mass index (BMI) is 16.2 (underweight).

14. a. Weight loss of 30 lb over 4 to 5 months, change in diet, and decreased appetite
    b. 24 oz of fluid/day; skin dry and flaky; fatigue; low BP; increased pulse and respirations; and voids four times a day, concentrated yellow urine
    c. Complaints of increasing fatigue

Chapter 9 Spiritual Assessment

1. Behavior: Praying
   Communication: Talking about God
   Relationships: Visits by clergy
   Environment: Religious objects such as a rosary, Bible, or Koran

2. Treatment, organ donation, abortion, dietary restrictions, gender of practitioner, and healing practices or rituals

3. Dietary constraints (e.g., Kosher diet)

4. Pro-life (antiabortion) viewpoint

5. May want same-sex practitioner; women may want to keep head covered; may refuse treatment because of fatalistic view

6. May wish to set up a small shrine in hospital room
7. May wish to use a crystal for healing potential
8. Mexican health practices encourage the use of a healer known as a curandero. Be aware of treatments prescribed by the healer, and evaluate them for any interactions with the patient's medical regimen.
9. People of Mexican heritage (usually Roman Catholic) often accept illness as a punishment from God for past sins. This belief may interfere with their seeking medical help or following a medical regimen. The patient's priest may help facilitate compliance with medical treatments.
10. She appears anxious and withdrawn, but when she speaks she says that her illness is a punishment. The religious symbols in her home and her use of rosary beads show that her spiritual life is important to her; however, she is in spiritual distress at present. You may need to assess further and intervene to help Mrs. Ramirez feel less anxious and more accepting of her illness and its treatment. Be sure to include her husband and the parish priest in your plan.

Chapter 10 Assessing the Integumentary System

1.

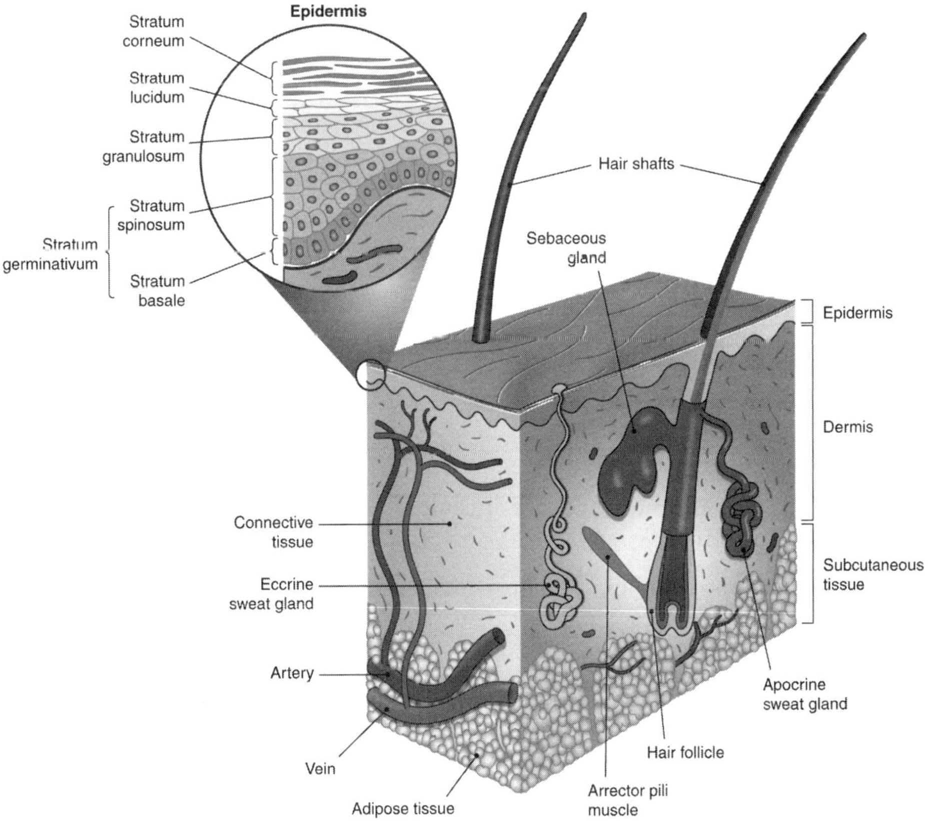

2. 1. c
   2. n
   3. f
   4. o
   5. g
   6. j
   7. h

8. l
9. k
10. m
11. a
12. i
13. b
14. e
15. d

3. Central cyanosis: Inspect oral mucosa or conjunctiva. Cyanosis indicates hypoxia. Peripheral cyanosis: Inspect nail bed. Cyanosis can be due to vasoconstriction or hypoxia.
4. The angle of attachment of the nail to the cuticle is greater than 180 degrees.
5. Do you have a history of skin cancer or other skin problems?
   Do you have a history of sun exposure?
   Do you have any medical problems, such as diabetes mellitus, cardiovascular disease, or endocrine problems?
   Do you have allergies?
   Are you on any medications? If so, what are they?
6. Size, shape, location, drainage, texture, pedunculation, color, and tenderness
7. Decreased skin elasticity, decreased sweat, atrophy and thinning of skin, and decreased pigmentation of skin and hair
8. Seborrheic keratosis, keratotic horns, actinic keratosis, and age spots
9. Asymmetry, border irregularity, color change or variegation, and diameter greater than 0.5 cm
10. Temperature, hydration, elasticity, color, and odor
11. Skin color changes may not be readily seen in dark skin, so assess the conjunctiva and oral mucosa for color changes.
12. Are you on any medications?
    Do you have any medical problems, such as thyroid disease?
    Have you recently been seriously ill?
    Do you have a family history of hair loss?
    Do you use hair dyes or have permanents?
13. For answers, see "Relationship of the Integumentary System to Other Systems," on page 210 of the text, and "Assessment of the Integumentary System's Relationship to Other Systems," on page 225 of the text.
14. Age, dementia, incontinence, and use of diapers, being bedridden, and restricted fluid intake
15. Frail, lethargic, inattentive; temperature 101.2°F; wrinkled, loose skin with poor turgor; stage 1 pressure ulcers on heels and sacrum; and dusky blue nails
16. Loose, wrinkled skin; poor skin turgor; gray hair; and increase in moles, cherry angiomas, and seborrheic keratosis
17. a. Stage 1 pressure ulcers on heels and sacrum, immobility, inattentive/confused, possible dehydration, and incontinence
    b. Restricted oral intake, temperature, poor skin turgor, and little urine output
    c. Incontinent, uses diapers, and confusion

19.

B	R	A	D	D	I	O	L	E	K	R	E
P	U	M	A	P	U	S	T	U	L	E	C
U	T	S	M	A	A	T	U	M	E	T	K
R	S	C	A	P	R	Y	M	O	S	E	P
U	M	A	C	U	L	E	O	S	I	K	Z
P	O	R	Y	T	P	C	R	C	O	T	S
K	L	E	S	E	R	O	S	I	O	N	M
T	E	U	T	S	U	R	C	R	U	S	T
E	R	P	U	R	P	U	R	A	P	U	T
T	S	Y	C	M	M	E	L	U	P	A	P

Chapter 11: Assessing the Head, Face, and Neck

1.

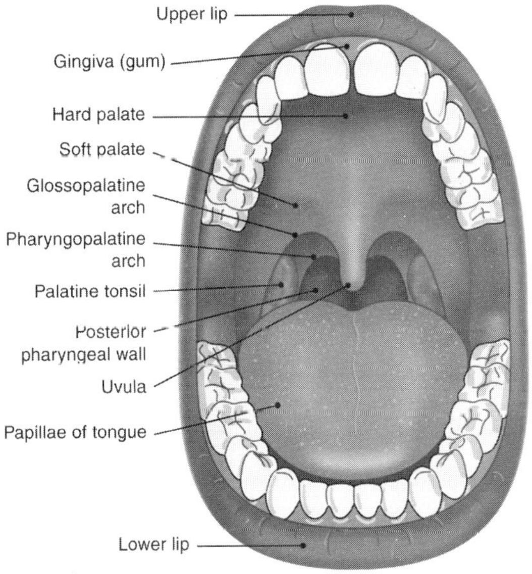

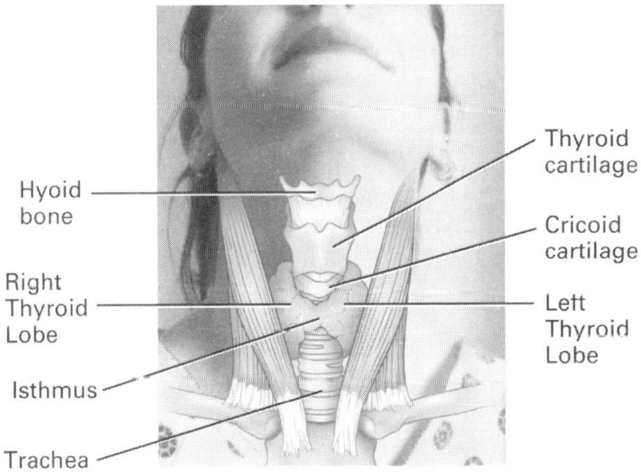

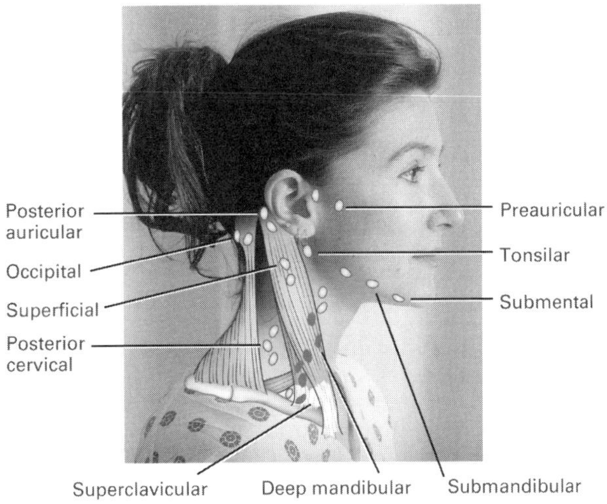

2. 1. b
   2. d
   3. g
   4. f
   5. j
   6. h
   7. c
   8. l
   9. i
   10. a
   11. e
   12. k
3. Red tonsils, exudates on tonsils, and enlarged tonsils
4. 20
5. Color, condition, and bite
6. Color, bleeding, and recession
7. Tetracycline, because it causes discoloration of teeth.
8.

Normal	Infection	Malignancy
≤1 cm	Enlarged	Enlarged
Round or oval	Round or oval	Irregular
Firm	Boggy	Hard
Movable	Movable	Fixed
Nontender	Tender	Nontender

9. Trapezius and sternocleidomastoid
10. Neutral, hyperextended, and as the person swallows
11. Below the cricoid cartilage
12. During pregnancy and puberty
13. Palpating fontanels and measuring head circumference
14. Nasolabial folds and palpebral fissures
15. For answers, see “Relationship of the Head, Face, and Neck to Other Systems,” on page 273 of the text, and “Assessment of the Head, Face, and Neck’s Relationship to Other Systems,” on page 313 of the text.
16. Communication problem related to slurred speech, risk for stroke, transient ischemic attack (TIA), family history of stroke, and risk for oral cancer related to history of smoking and chewing tobacco and positive family history of oral cancer
17. HTN, TIA, carotid bruits, positive family history, being slightly overweight, and eating fried foods
18. Speech difficulty, paralysis in right extremities, urinary incontinence, BP 186/108 mm Hg, decreased muscle strength on left side 4/5, movements clumsy, positive carotid bruits, and asymmetry of facial features
19. Positive family history, positive smoking history and use of chewing tobacco, positive oral lesion and enlarged submandibular nodes, and weight loss
20. Diet, HTN, stroke, oral cancer, and chewing tobacco

21. a. Decreased motor function on left side of face, oral lesion, and unexplained weight loss
    b. Risk for aspiration
    c. Slurred speech

23. 1. S (K) U L L
    2. T H Y R (O) I D
    3. U V U (L) A
    4. S I N (U) S E S
    5. C R (I) C O I D
    6. T O N S I (L) S
    7. T U R B I N (A) T E S
    8. L Y M (P) H
    9. T (E) E T H
    10. G I N G I V (A)
    11. N E C (K)
    12. G O I T E R

    K O L U I L A P E A K
    A precancerous oral lesion is called LEUKOPLAKIA.

Chapter 12: Assessing the Eye and the Ear

The Eye

1.

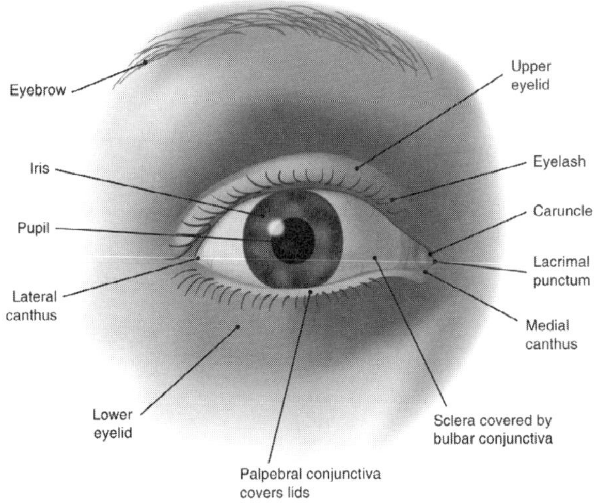

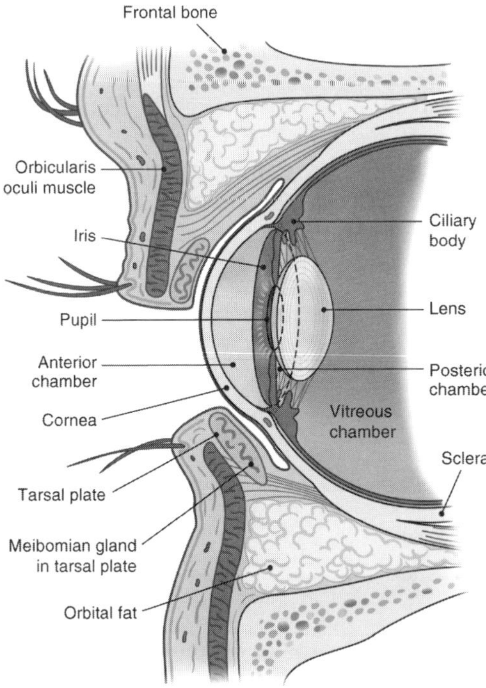

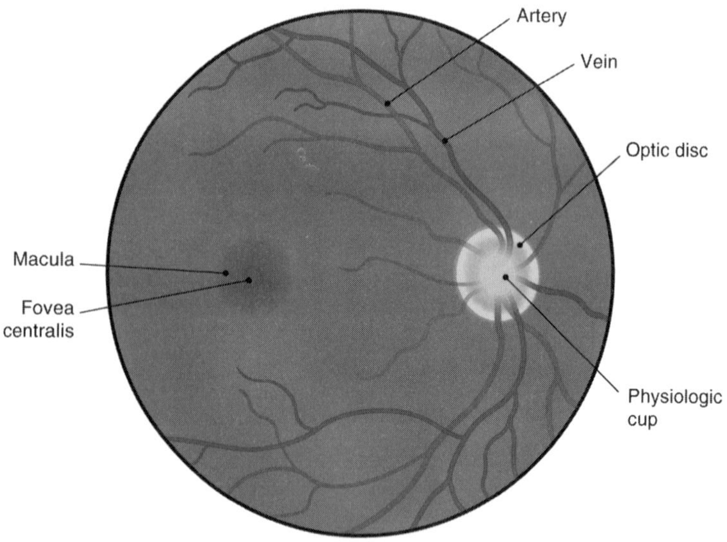

Right eye

2. 1. f
   2. n
   3. d
   4. e
   5. m
   6. j
   7. k
   8. b
   9. c
   10. h
   11. a
   12. i
   13. g
   14. l

3. OD 20/50: He can see at 20 feet what someone with normal far vision (20/20) could see at 50 feet with the right eye.
   OS 20/40: He can see at 20 feet what someone with normal far vision could see at 40 feet with the left eye.
   OU 20/40: He can see at 20 feet what someone with normal far vision could see at 40 feet with both eyes.

4. No. Normal 20/20 vision is usually attained by the time the child reaches school age.

5. Six cardinal fields of gaze test, cover-uncover test, and corneal light reflex test

6. 1. c
   2. a
   3. b
   4. e
   5. d
   6. g
   7. f

7. Darken the room, examine same eye to same eye, have the patient look straight ahead, and always examine the macula last.

8. a. Used for undilated pupil
   b. Used for dilated pupil
   c. Used with fluorescein dye
   d. Filters red
   e. Locates lesions
   f. Used to determine shape of lesion

9. For answers, see "Relationship of the Eyes to Other Systems," on pages 327 and 368 of the text, and "Assessment of the Eyes' Relationship to Other Systems," on pages 340 and 386 of the text.

10. What medications are you taking? She should not take mydriatic-producing medications because they dilate the pupil and increase intraocular pressure.

11. Tonometry

12. Blindness

13. Her race—Incidence of glaucoma is higher in African-Americans than in other races.

14. a. Complaint of severe eye pain
    b. Decreased peripheral vision and blurred vision
    c. Blurred vision, decreased peripheral vision, and colored halos

16.

1.	S	(C)	L	E	R	A							
2.	I	R	I	S									
3.	(M)	E	D	I	A	L	C	A	N	T	H	U	S
4.	C	O	R	N	E	A							
5.	(L)	A	C	R	I	M	A	L	G	L	A	N	D
6.	R	E	T	I	N	A							
7.	C	O	N	J	U	N	C	T	I	V	(A)		
8.	P	(U)	P	I	L								
9.	L	E	N	S									
10.	F	O	V	E	(A)								

C M L A U A
Always examine the MACULA last on funduscopic examination.

The Ear

1.

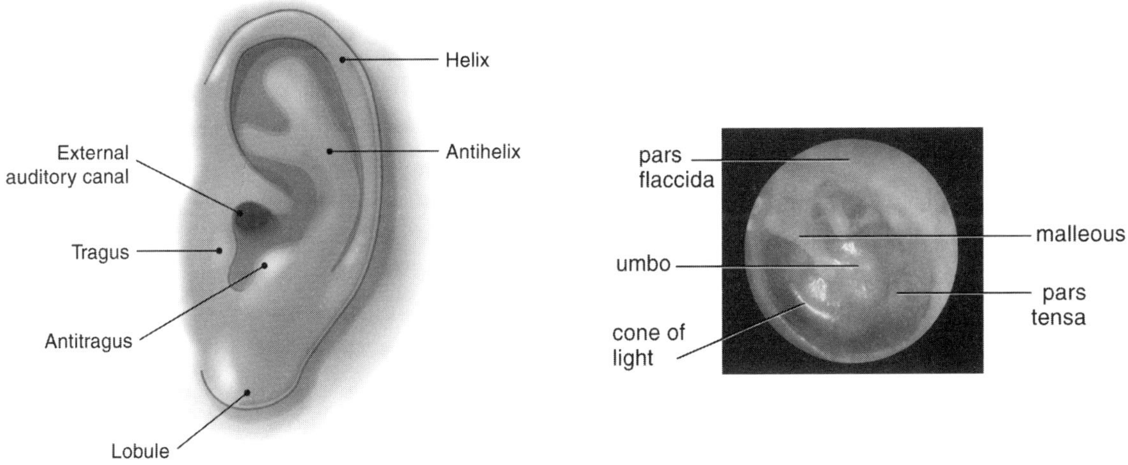

2. 1. c
   2. d
   3. h
   4. g
   5. a
   6. b
   7. e
   8. f

3. Do you have a history of frequent ear infections?
   Are you taking any medications?
   Have you ever had trauma to your ears?
   Do you have a family history of hearing problems?
   Are you exposed to noise pollution?

4. With conductive hearing loss, the sound lateralizes to the bad ear. With sensorineural hearing loss, the sound lateralizes to the good ear.

5. AC > BC; AC < BC

6. Bloody drainage: Trauma
   Purulent drainage: Infection
   Clear/serous drainage: Allergies or cerebrospinal fluid (CSF)

7. Tragus, mastoid, and helix (pull forward)

8. Young child: Pull ear canal down.
   Adult: Pull ear canal up and back.

9. Color of tympanic membrane and external ear canal, position of landmarks, intactness of drum, and mobility of drum

10. In a young child, the shape, size, and position of the ear canal and eustachian tubes—shorter, wider, and more horizontal—increase the risk for infection.

11. For answers, see "Relationship of the Eyes and the Ears to Other Systems," on pages 327 and 368 of the text, and "Assessment of the Eyes' and the Ears' Relationship to Other Systems," on pages 340 and 386 of the text.

12. Age, gender, history of recurrent ear infection, recent upper respiratory infection, and family history of otitis media

13. Exposure to second-hand smoke and bottle-feeding

14. Mobility of the drum

15. a. Brian's complaint that "my ear hurts," tugging at ear, irritability, and tenderness of external ear
    b. Recurrent ear infections
    c. Fever and not eating well
    d. Pain and not sleeping well

17. 1. O T I Ⓣ I S M Ⓔ D I A
    2. T Ⓡ A G U S
    3. M A S T O Ⓘ D
    4. I Ⓝ C U S
    5. M A L L Ⓔ O L U S

6. S T (A) P E S
7. C (O) C H L E A
8. H E (L) I (X)
9. E X O (S) (T) O S I S
10. C H O L E S (T) E A T O M A

TERINEAOLXISTT
Another name for swimmer's ear is EXTERNAL OTITIS.

Chapter 13 Assessing the Respiratory System

1.

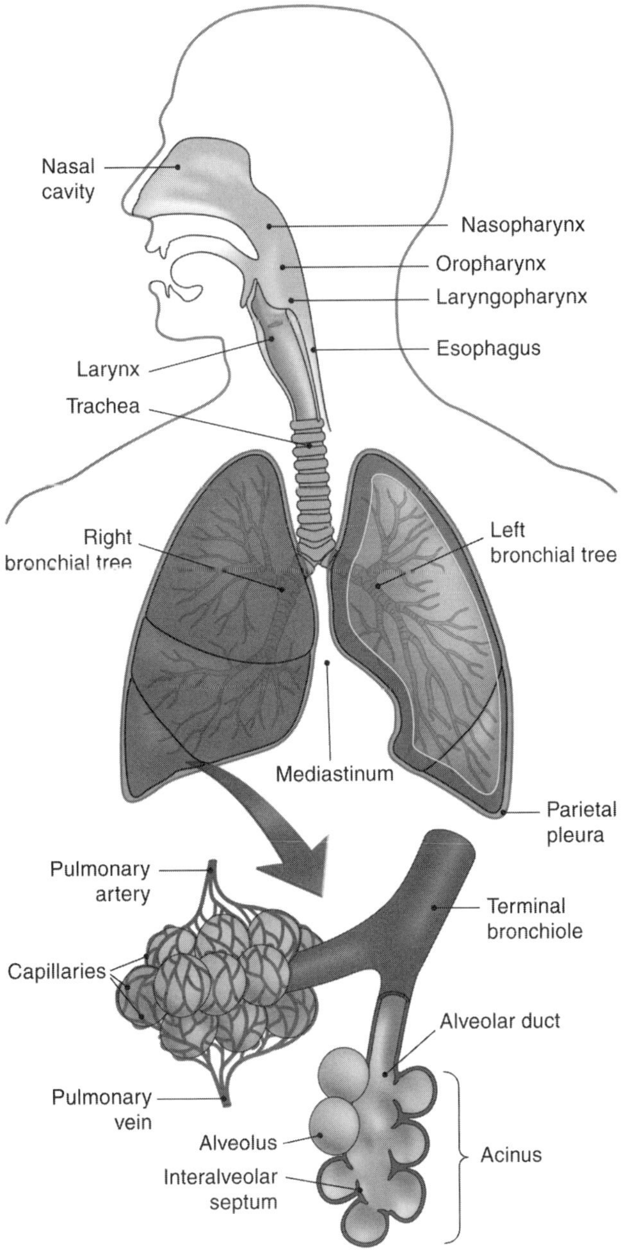

2. 1. c
   2. e
   3. f
   4. b
   5. a
   6. d

3. 1. j
   2. d
   3. i
   4. g
   5. c
   6. b
   7. a
   8. e
   9. h
   10. f

4. Decreased breath sounds resulting from poor ventilatory effort, and shape of chest (e.g., musculoskeletal changes associated with aging)

5. Peripheral cyanosis occurs in the periphery as a result of a localized problem or vasoconstriction. Central cyanosis results from hypoxia and is seen not only in the extremities but also in the oral mucosa and conjunctiva.

6. Change in mental status, confusion, or agitation

7. Bronchial breath sounds over the affected lung with some crackles and rhonchi

8. The right middle lobe is anatomically situated so that it can be assessed only from the anterior or lateral approach.

9. Neurologic system: Changes in mental status, such as confusion, irritability, and agitation
   Integumentary system: Skin color changes, such as duskiness, pallor, or cyanosis; clammy skin
   Cardiovascular system: Increased pulse rate and vasoconstriction

10. For answers, see "Relationship of the Respiratory System to Other Systems," on page 397 of the text, and "Assessment of the Respiratory System's Relationship to Other Systems," on page 419 of the text.

11. Upper respiratory infection

12. Right congestive heart failure secondary to emphysema

13. Signs/symptoms of hypoxia, including fatigue, shortness of breath, and central and peripheral cyanosis

14. Emphysema can cause overinflation of lungs, which pushes diaphragm down to T12. Because lungs are overinflated, no change is seen when assessing diaphragmatic excursion.

15. Barrel chest, costal angle greater than 90 degrees, pursed-lip breathing, shortness of breath, hyperresonance at bases, level of diaphragm at T12, and decreased breath sounds at bases

16. a. Productive cough, foul-smelling yellow mucus, shortness of breath, respirations 28/min, and scattered rhonchi and wheezes
    b. Shortness of breath, difficulty moving secretions, clubbing, pale gray mucous membranes, and reduced activity tolerance
    c. Shortness of breath, decreased appetite, and being underweight

18.

Y	Y	N	O	H	P	O	L	B	Y
L	L	O	B	E	B	W	H	I	Y
W	U	T	R	A	C	H	E	A	N
I	N	E	O	P	W	E	E	R	O
E	G	O	N	P	H	E	E	A	H
U	L	U	C	G	E	Z	Z	C	P
E	V	W	H	E	E	Z	E	H	O
V	E	S	I	C	U	L	A	R	G
U	T	R	A	S	T	H	M	A	E
A	S	A	L	V	E	O	L	I	B

Chapter 14 Assessing the Cardiovascular System

1.

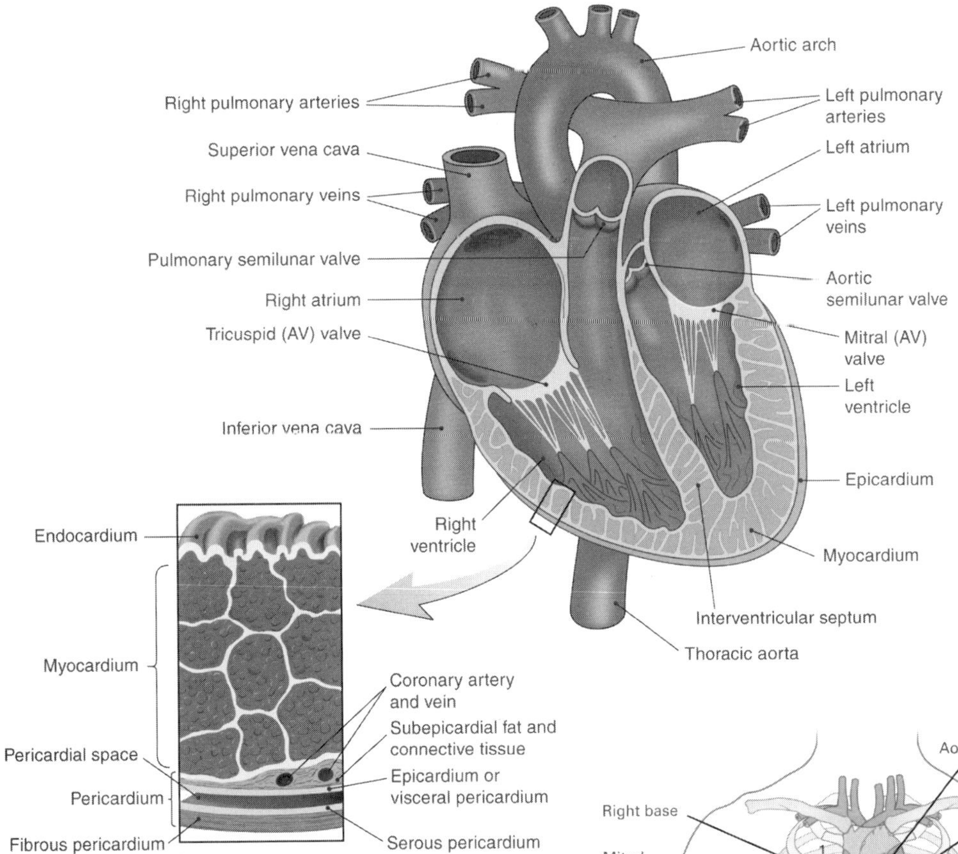

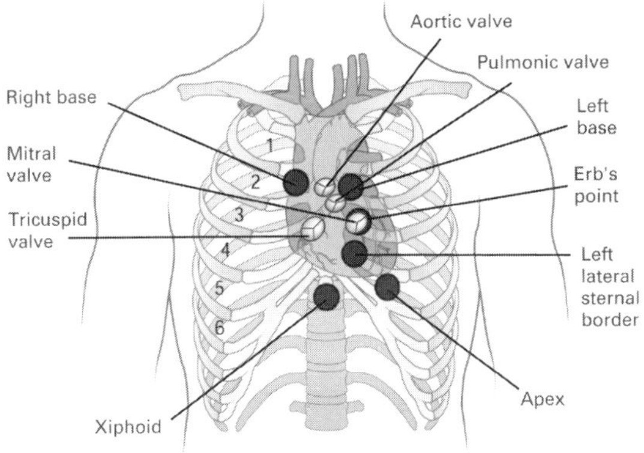

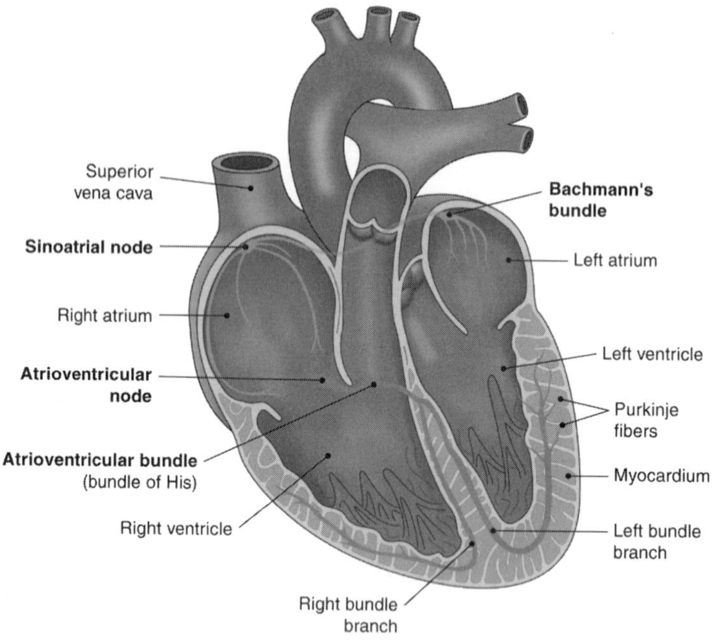

2. 1. f
   2. g
   3. e
   4. o
   5. m
   6. b
   7. h
   8. c
   9. a
   10. i
   11. l
   12. n
   13. j
   14. k
   15. d

3. 1. c
   2. g
   3. h
   4. i
   5. b
   6. j
   7. e
   8. f
   9. d
   10. a

4. S_1 is louder at the apex; S_2 is louder at the base.

5. Split S_1 at tricuspid area; split S_2 at pulmonic area

6. During inspiration, more blood returns to the right side of the heart than the left side. This means that the right side of the heart takes more time to pump, resulting in a split S_2 during inspiration.

7. S_1 is loudest at apex; S_2 is loudest at base.
   S_1 correlates with QRS of ECG.
   S_1 precedes palpable carotid pulsation.
8. S_4: Late diastolic sound heard when left atrium contracts against resistance.
9. S_3: Early diastolic sound heard as blood rushes into a dilated, noncompliant left ventricle.
10. Carotid pulsation is palpable; jugular pulsation is not.
    Carotids have one upstroke; jugulars have an undulated wave.
    Carotids are not affected by position; jugulars are.
    Carotids are not affected by respirations; jugulars are.
11. The sternal angle (angle of Louis) and the highest point of jugular venous pulsation
12. a. Split S_1 from S_4: Split S_1 is a high-pitched systolic sound heard best at the left lower sternal border. An S_4 is a low-pitched diastolic sound heard best at the apex.
    b. Split S_1 from ejection click: Split S_1 is a high-pitched systolic sound heard best at the left lower sternal border. An ejection click is a high-pitched mid-to-late systolic sound.
    c. Split S_2 from S_3: Split S_2 is a high-pitched systolic sound heard best at base left during inspiration. S_3 is a low-pitched diastolic sound heard best at the apex.
    d. Split S_2 from opening snap: Split S_2 is a high-pitched diastolic sound heard best at base left during inspiration. An opening snap is a high-pitched diastolic sound heard best at the apex.
13. Pericardial friction rub—A high-pitched, scratchy sound heard best at the left lower sternal border
14. Increased flow through a normal valve, flow through a constricted valve, flow into a dilated chamber, shunting, and backflow through an incompetent valve
15. Location heard, pitch, duration, quality, timing in cardiac cycle, and intensity
16. Diastolic murmur or murmur greater than grade 3
17. Have patient hold breath; the bell.
18. For answers, see "Relationship of the Cardiovascular System to Other Systems," on page 452 of the text, and "Assessment of the Cardiovascular System's Relationship to Other Systems," on page 467 of the text.
19. Cardiovascular and respiratory
20. HTN and left ventricular hypertrophy
21. Signs of right-sided heart failure
22. S_4 could be associated with HTN or acute myocardial infarction, and S_3 could be associated with congestive heart failure.
23. a. Complains of chest discomfort; anxious, clutching chest; and elevated BP, pulse, and respirations
    b. Appears anxious; states, "Am I going to die?"; and has increase in vital signs
    c. Skin pale/ashen and diaphoretic; mucous membranes pale gray; capillary refill poor; skin cool, pale, shiny, and hairless on lower extremities; and +1 peripheral pulses
    d. Tachycardia with irregular rhythm; HTN; ECG shows anterior wall myocardial infarction, S_3, and S_4; skin ashen, cool, and diaphoretic; poor capillary refill; bibasilar crackles; neck vein distension and jugular venous pressure greater than 3 cm; and positive abdominal jugular reflux
24. Decreased cardiac output and ineffective tissue perfusion. Improving cardiac output and tissue perfusion is essential to maintain life.

26.

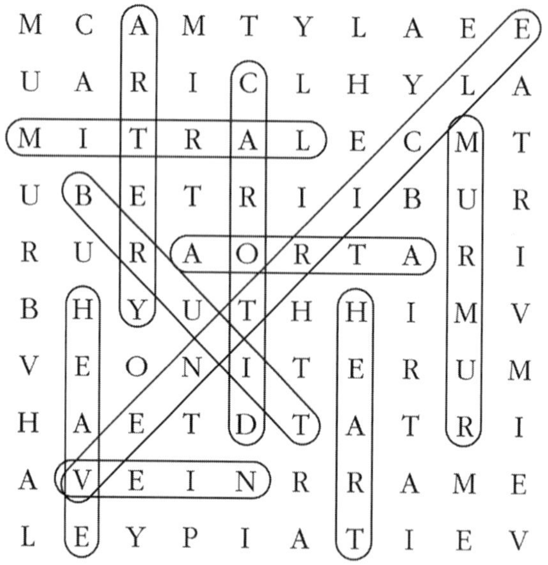

Chapter 15: Assessing the Peripheral-Vascular and Lymphatic Systems

1.

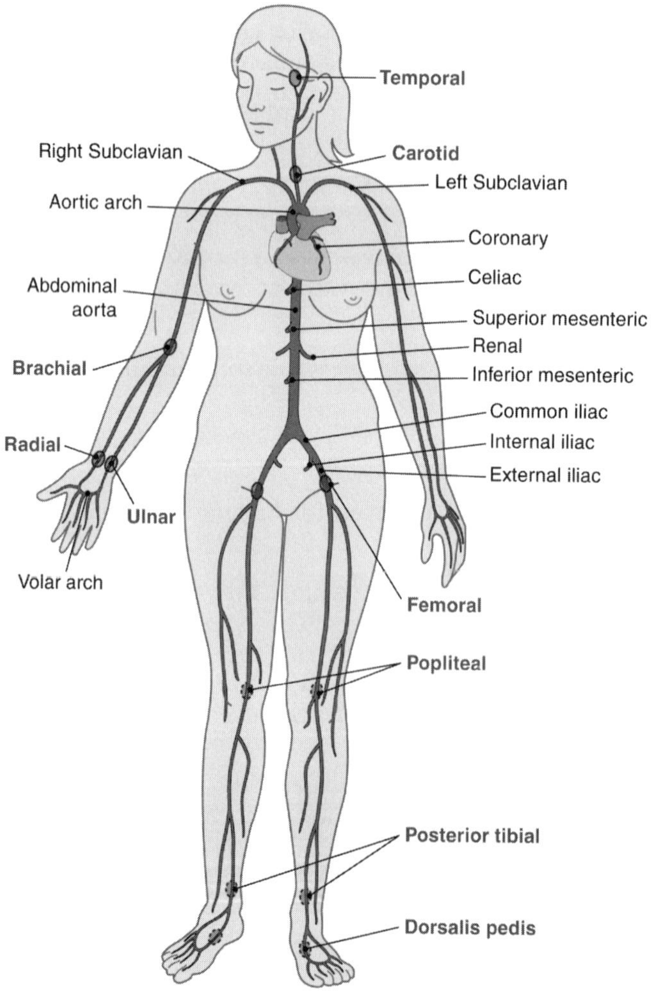

2. 1. c
   2. f
   3. e
   4. j
   5. d
   6. b
   7. h
   8. i
   9. a
   10. g

3. As you inflate the cuff, palpate the brachial artery to the point at which the pulse is obliterated, then deflate the cuff. Reinflate the cuff 20 to 30 mm higher than the point at which the pulse was obliterated, and listen for BP.

4. Supine, sitting, and standing

5. BP: Systolic pressure drops 20 mm Hg.
   Pulse: Pulse rate increases about 20 BPM.
   Level of consciousness: Patient feels light-headed or faint.

6. Rate, rhythm, contour, elasticity, amplitude, and equality

7. Decreased elasticity

8. Arterial insufficiency: Absent or decreased pulse; pallor or rubor; thin, hairless skin; and lesions on toes
   Venous insufficiency: Edema; brownish discoloration; thick, leathery skin; and lesions on ankles

9. Ankle-brachial index

10. Size, shape, consistency, tenderness, and mobility

11. Enlarged, round, boggy-to-firm, tender, mobile nodes

12. Lymph nodes are biggest in childhood and get smaller with age.

13. For answers, see "Relationship of the Lymphatic System to Other Systems," on page 496 of the text, and "Assessment of the Lymphatic System's Relationship to Other Systems," on page 507 of the text.

14. History of HTN, diabetes mellitus, coronary artery disease, and smoking; family history of myocardial infarction and stroke

15. Lesions on toes; absent pulses; thin, shiny skin on extremities, with patchy hair loss; thick nails; color changes in legs; and cool feet

16. Ankle-brachial index

17. Because blood flow must be adequate to the lower extremities to ensure healing.

18. a. Intermittent claudication and cramping in legs when walking, relieved by rest
    b. Intermittent claudication; cool feet; absent pedal pulses; thin, shiny skin and patchy hair loss on extremities; and color changes in legs
    c. Ulcers on toes

20. Diet, vascular disease, diabetes mellitus, HTN, and foot care

21. Walking exercises for 15 to 30 minutes several times a day to improve collateral circulation

22. Inspect feet daily, do not soak feet, keep feet clean and dry, wear shoes that fit properly, and have podiatrist cut toenails.

23.

1.	(B)	R	A	C	H	I	A	L								
2.	K	O	R	O	(T)	K	O	F	F							
3.	B	U	E	(R)	G	E	R'	S	D	I	S	E	A	S	E	
4.	R	A	Y	N	A	(U)	D'	S	D	I	(S)	E	A	S	E	
5.	H	O	M	A	N	S'	S	(I)	G	N						
6.	A	L	L	E	N	T	E	S	T							
7.	P	O	P	L	I	T	E	A	L							
8.	F	E	M	O	R	A	L									
9.	V	E	I	N												
10.	A	R	T	E	R	Y										

B T R U S I

Arteries are auscultated for BRUITS.

Chapter 16 Assessing the Breasts

1.

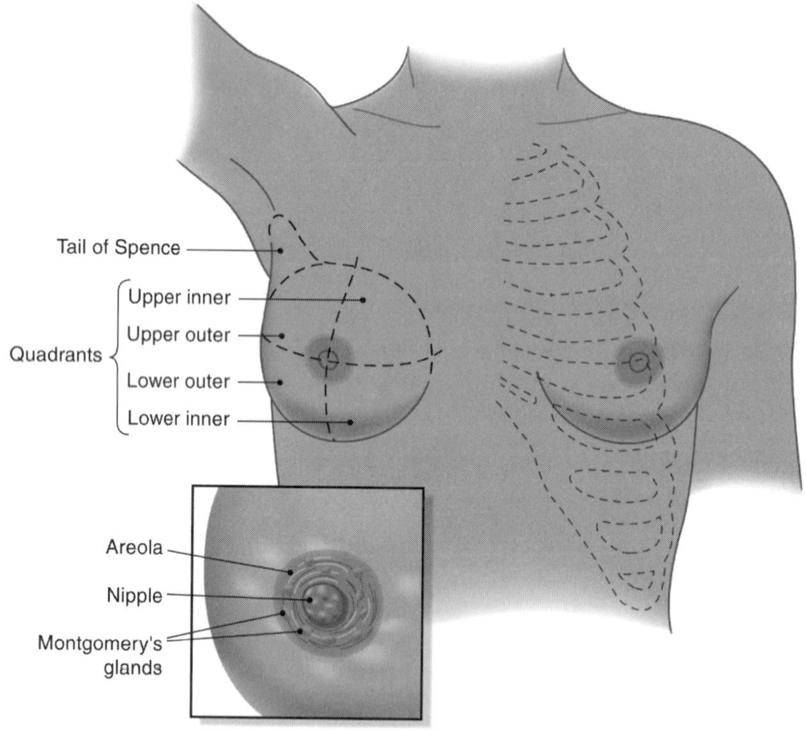

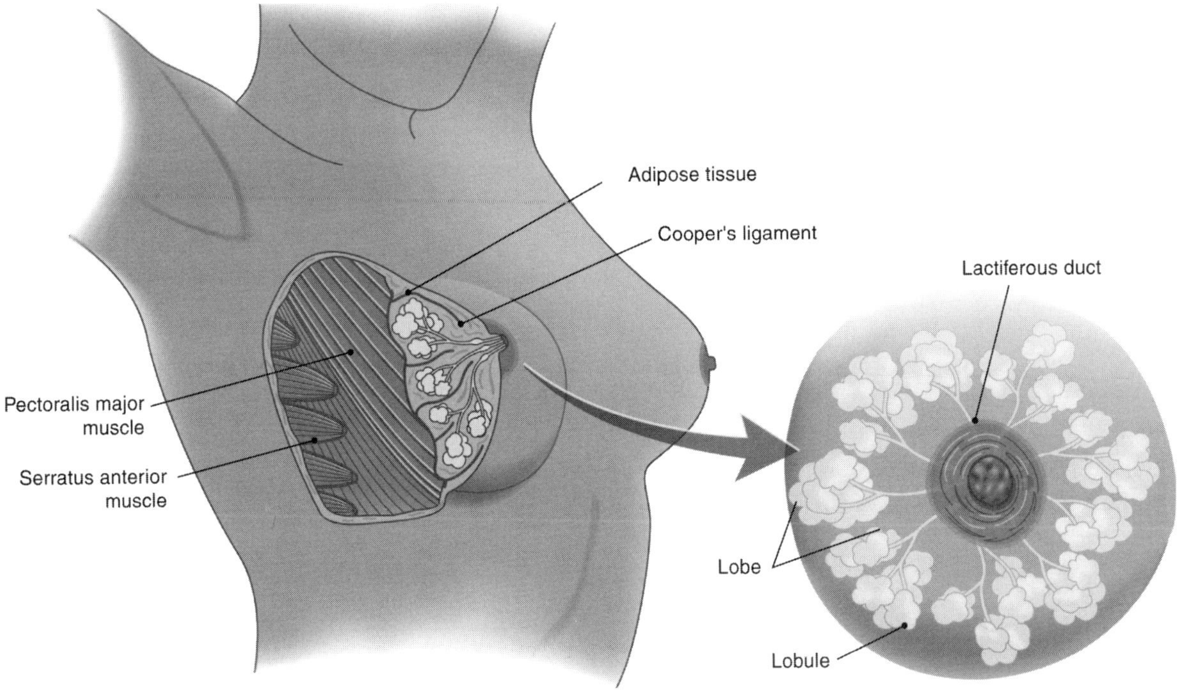

2. 1. c
   2. d
   3. b
   4. e
   5. a
3. Have you ever had breast cancer?
   Do you have a family history of breast cancer?
   Are you childless, or did you have your first child after age 30?
4. On the 5th to 7th day of her menstrual cycle
5. Sitting with hands at sides; sitting with hands over head; sitting with hands on hips; and standing, leaning forward
6. Size, shape, consistency, mobility, and tenderness
7. Increase in breast size and a mass that is hard, irregular in shape, and nonmobile and nontender
8. 1. c
   2. d
   3. a
   4. b
9. For answers, see "Relationship of the Breasts to Other Systems," on page 531 of the text, and "Assessment of the Breasts' Relationship to Other Systems," on page 542 of the text.
10. Age, family history, race, early menarche, first full-term pregnancy after age 30
11. Lymph nodes

12. a. Scheduled for lumpectomy.
b. Anxious, nervous, and tearful; states, "I'm so afraid it might be cancer."
c. Scheduled for lumpectomy.

14. 1. P A G (E) T' S
2. M (A) S (T) I T I S
3. (F) I B R (O) A D E N O M A
4. A R (E) O (L) A
5. N (I) P (P) L E
6. A (C) I N I
7. G Y (N) E C O M A (S) T I A

E A T F O E L I P C N S
The most frequent site of breast cancer in women is the TAIL OF SPENCE.

Chapter 17 Assessing the Abdomen

1.

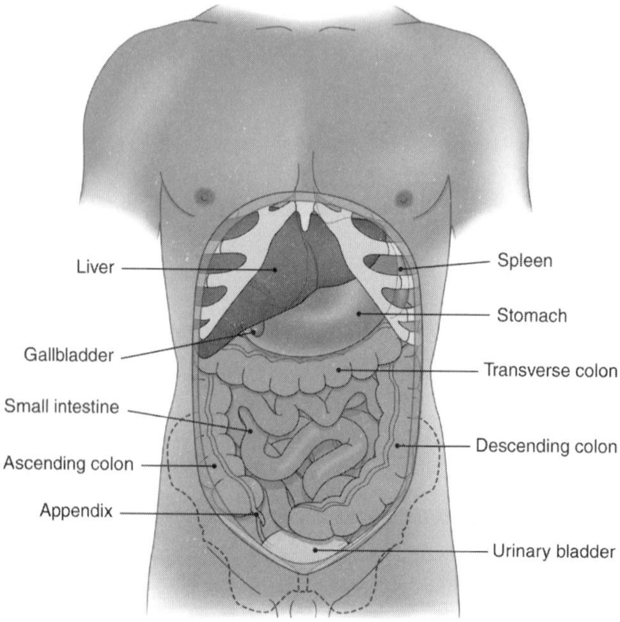

2. 1. b
2. d
3. a
4. c
5. f
6. e
7. j
8. g
9. i
10. h

3. Liver: Right upper quadrant
Gallbladder: Right upper quadrant
Pancreas: Right upper quadrant and left upper quadrant
Stomach: Left upper quadrant

Spleen: Left upper quadrant
Cecum: Right lower quadrant
Appendix: Right lower quadrant
Sigmoid colon: Left lower quadrant
Transverse colon: Right upper quadrant, right lower quadrant, and left upper quadrant
Ascending colon: Right upper quadrant
Descending colon: Left upper quadrant and left lower quadrant

4. 1. c
   2. a
   3. d
   4. e
   5. b

5. Respirations, aortic pulsations, and peristalsis

6. Palpation could alter bowel sounds.

7. 5 minutes

8. Location: Right lower quadrant
   Rationale: Active site; connects small and large intestine

9. Effects of anesthesia, abdominal surgery, and decreased mobility

10. Pain medication and immobility

11. Diarrhea and early obstruction

12. Scratch test

13. Dullness

14. 6 to 12 cm

15. No, the spleen needs to be about three times its normal size to be palpable.

16. Midaxillary line

17. For answers, see "Relationship of GI to Other Systems," on page 560 of the text, and "Assessment of the Abdomen's Relationship to Other Systems," on page 582 of the text.

18. A response to the pain. Shallow breathing minimizes abdominal movement.

19. Time of last meal influences types of anesthesia or need for nasogastric tube to prevent aspiration if surgery is necessary.

20. Do you have any allergies to drugs (e.g., penicillin), food, environmental factors, or latex?

21. Temperature elevation: Inflammatory response, infection
    Increased respirations: Response to pain

22. Temperature elevation; increased, shallow respirations; guarding; decreased bowel sounds; tenderness in right lower quadrant; positive iliopsoas, Rovsing's, rebound, and obturator signs; cutaneous hypersensitivity signs; and body posture

23. a. Statement of level 10 pain in abdomen; guarding abdomen; shallow, increased respiratory rate; and high-normal range on pulse, temperature, and BP
    b. Statement about nausea and vomiting at home
    c. Nausea, vomiting, and temperature elevation

24. Apply ice bag to painful area, give nothing by mouth (NPO) in anticipation of upcoming surgery, give pain medications as ordered, and place patient in semi-Fowler's position so that abdominal drainage can collect in lower quadrants.

25. Muscle rigidity over entire abdomen; elevated BP, pulse, respiratory rate, and temperature; states that abdominal pain is worse with movement and coughing and better when flexing right hip and knee; abdomen is rigid or boardlike; bowel sounds are diminished.

27.
1. L I V E **R**
2. **P** E R I S T A L S I S
3. **S** **T** R I A E
4. **M** E L E N A
5. F L A T **U** S
6. **C** H Y M E
7. B O R **B** O R **Y** G M I
8. A S C I T E S
9. D I A R R H **E** A
10. M A S T I C A T I **O** **N**
11. S P L E E **N**
12. C **I** R R H O S I S

R P S T M U C B Y E O N N I
The area of tenderness in acute appendicitis is MCBURNEY'S POINT.

Chapter 18 Assessing the Female Genitourinary System

1.

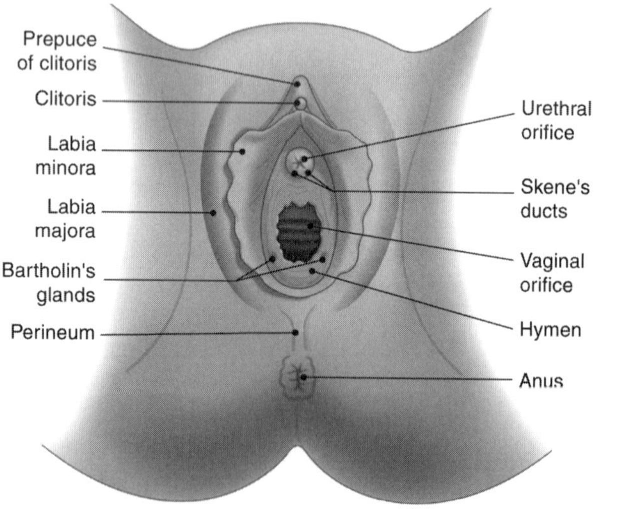

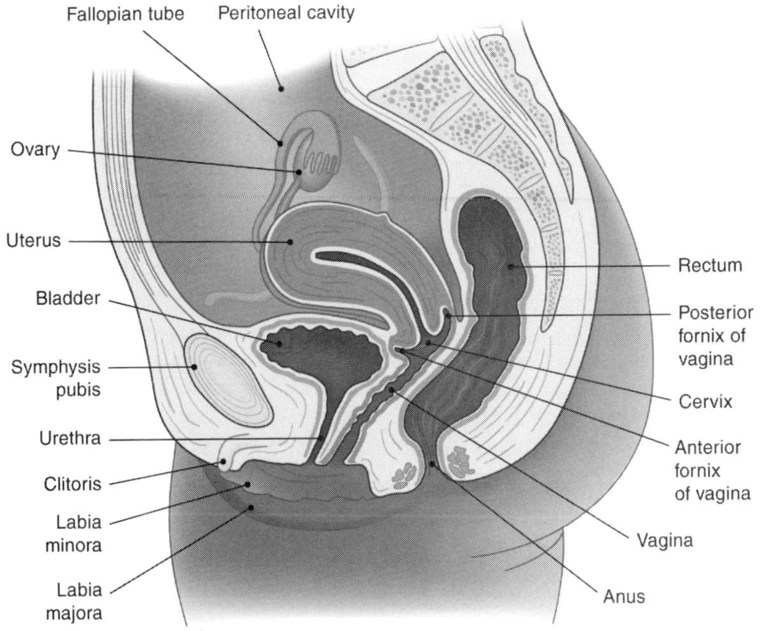

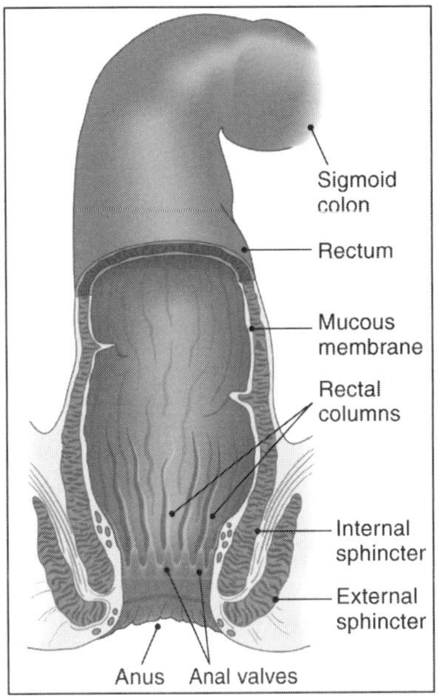

2.
    1. g
    2. f
    3. h
    4. i
    5. j
    6. d
    7. k
    8. l
    9. c
    10. e
    11. b
    12. a

3. Decreased, irregular, or absent menses; hot flashes; and decreased vaginal secretions

4. At age 21, or 3 years after becoming sexually active

5. A test for cervical cancer

6. At what age did your menstrual periods start?
   Can you describe your cycle? How often do you menstruate? How many days per month?
   How much do you bleed?
   Do you use pads or tampons?
   Are you sexually active?
   If yes, do you practice safe sex? Do you use birth control?

7. 16 years

8. To assess the reproductive organs (uterus, ovaries, cervix, and vagina), to detect any lesions, and to obtain specimens

9. Parous: Os appears as a slit.
   Nulliparous: Os appears round and closed.

10.
1. b
2. f
3. e
4. a
5. h
6. j
7. k
8. l
9. m
10. g
11. c
12. d
13. i

11. For answers, see "Relationship of the Female Genitourinary System to Other Systems" on page 616 of the text and "Assessment of the Female Genitourinary System," on page 635 of the text.

12. Vague abdominal complaints, change in bowel habits, loss of appetite, and weight loss but increase in abdominal girth

13. Menarche age 11, nulliparous, age and race, fatty diet, and family history of ovarian cancer

14. The respiratory system because ascites may push up the diaphragm and impinge respirations

15. a. Progressive vague abdominal complaints.
b. Change in bowel pattern; reports constipation.
c. Affect anxious; states she is "scared about what the doctor will find."

16. a. Surgical incision is a break in skin, the first line of defense.
b. Ascites may push diaphragm up and impinge respirations. Anesthesia may lead to hypoventilation. Pain may lead to hypoventilation.

18.

B	C	P	A	Y	M	P	U	M	L
L	E	V	R	A	E	U	R	E	P
A	R	A	R	N	N	B	E	N	A
D	V	X	E	I	S	L	T	A	R
O	I	A	C	G	E	A	H	R	I
D	X	G	R	A	S	D	R	C	T
E	G	R	A	V	I	D	A	H	Y
R	T	U	R	E	T	E	R	E	G
R	A	P	U	B	E	R	T	Y	H
C	L	A	P	R	M	E	N	S	L

Chapter 19 Assessing the Male Genitourinary System

1.

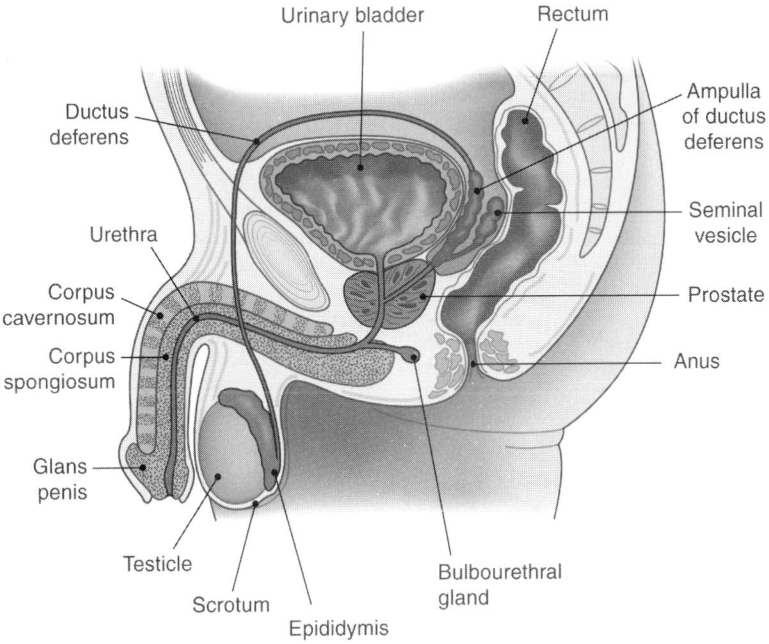

2. 1. f
   2. g
   3. j
   4. b
   5. k
   6. e
   7. a
   8. d
   9. c
   10. h
   11. i

3. 1. c
   2. j
   3. a
   4. l
   5. d
   6. h
   7. e
   8. i
   9. g
   10. b
   11. f
   12. k

4. Risk factors are cryptorchidism and exposure to diethylstilbestrol (DES).
Testicular self-exam (TSE) should be done monthly.
Testicles should be egg-shaped and feel rubbery, firm, mobile, and nontender.

5. Age 50
   Prostatic-specific antigen test and digital rectal examination
6. Alcohol and drug abuse, smoking, medications, and medical problems such as diabetes and cardiovascular disease
7. Indirect and direct inguinal hernias and femoral hernias
8. For answers, see "Relationship of the Male Genitourinary System to Other Systems," on page 655 of the text, and "Assessment of the Male Genitourinary System's Relationship to Other Systems," on page 666 of the text.
9. Maintain open line of communication and remain nonjudgmental.
   Determine through questioning what patient knows about human immunodeficiency virus (HIV) and other sexually transmitted diseases (STDs).
   Perform physical exam.
   Obtain STD screening tests and HIV test, explaining limitations of tests.
   Discuss possible outcomes and potential interventions.
   Provide education about STD prevention.
10. Multiple sex partners, frequent sex with inconsistent use of condoms, excessive alcohol use, marijuana use, and history of STDs
11. Condyloma (human papillomavirus)
12. Use of condoms, types of STDs, and drug and alcohol use
13. a. Unprotected sexual activity, drug and alcohol use, and multiple sex partners
    b. Unprotected sexual activity, multiple partners, and risky behavior with drugs and alcohol
    c. Unprotected sexual activity and multiple partners

15.

S	N	O	I	T	C	E	R	E	P
E	C	E	J	A	C	U	T	A	E
H	E	R	N	I	A	S	E	M	N
S	C	R	O	T	U	M	A	C	I
P	R	O	S	T	A	T	E	P	S
E	J	A	C	U	L	A	T	E	U
R	I	N	S	S	E	M	E	N	L
M	U	R	E	T	H	R	A	I	A
P	E	R	S	S	E	T	S	E	T
H	E	R	N	I	S	P	E	R	E

Chapter 20 Assessing the Musculoskeletal System

1. 1. e
   2. c
   3. d
   4. g
   5. f
   6. a
   7. b

2. a. Hinge
   b. Ball and socket
   c. Condyloid
   d. Gliding/plane
   e. Hinge
   f. Ball and socket
   g. Saddle

3. 1. d
   2. h
   3. b
   4. l
   5. m
   6. c
   7. j
   8. e
   9. f
   10. k
   11. a
   12. i
   13. g

4. Standing and bending over, or "dive" position

5. Cervical, thoracic, lumbar, and sacral

6. Kyphosis: Accentuated thoracic curve
   Scoliosis: Lateral deviation of spine
   Lordosis: Accentuated lumbar curve

7. Arm length: Measure from acromium process to tip of middle finger
   Leg length: Measure from anterior superior iliac crest to medial malleolus

8. Back pain, gait problem, and an apparent scoliosis

9. If right arm is dominant side, circumference may be greater because of activity, such as sports.

10. Stride length, base of support, conformity of phases, arm swing, toe position, and cadence

11. Short stride length, wide base of support, and problems with phases (e.g., swing phase cadence may not be rhythmic).

12. Wide base of support and shortened stride length

13. Kyphosis

14. ROM, deformity, redness, swelling, crepitus, pain, and stability

15. 5 = Normal; 4 = movement against some resistance; 3 = movement against gravity with no resistance.

16. Observe gait; have patient hop on one foot, tandem walk (heel to toe), heel-and-toe walk, and do deep knee bends; and perform Romberg's test.

17. Upper: Rapid alternating movements and finger-thumb opposition
    Lower: Toe tapping and heel down shin

18. Point-to-point localization and finger to nose

19. For answers, see "Relationship of the Musculoskeletal System to Other Systems," on page 692 of the text, and "Assessment of the Relationship of the Musculoskeletal System to Other Systems," on page 704 of the text.

20. Age, weight, and occupation

21. Her occupation

22. a. Pain in lower back when sitting or lying for extended periods. "Feels like a dull knife in my lower back, I usually get up and walk around to relieve it. It's my bones; they are getting old." Rates pain as 7 on 1-to-10 scale. Diagnosed with DJD 2 years ago, which has been getting progressively worse.
    b. Cannot sit or stand for prolonged periods without developing pain.

24. 1. B O N (E)
    2. (T) E N D O N
    3. L (I) G A M E (N) T
    4. (L) U M B A R
    5. S (P) I N E
    6. B A L A (N) C E
    7. S A C R A (L)
    8. T (H) O R A C I C
    9. G (A) I T
    10. M U S C L (E)

    E T I N L P N L H A E
    Two tests for carpal tunnel syndrome are the TINEL and PHALEN tests.

Chapter 21: Assessing the Sensory-Neurologic System

1.

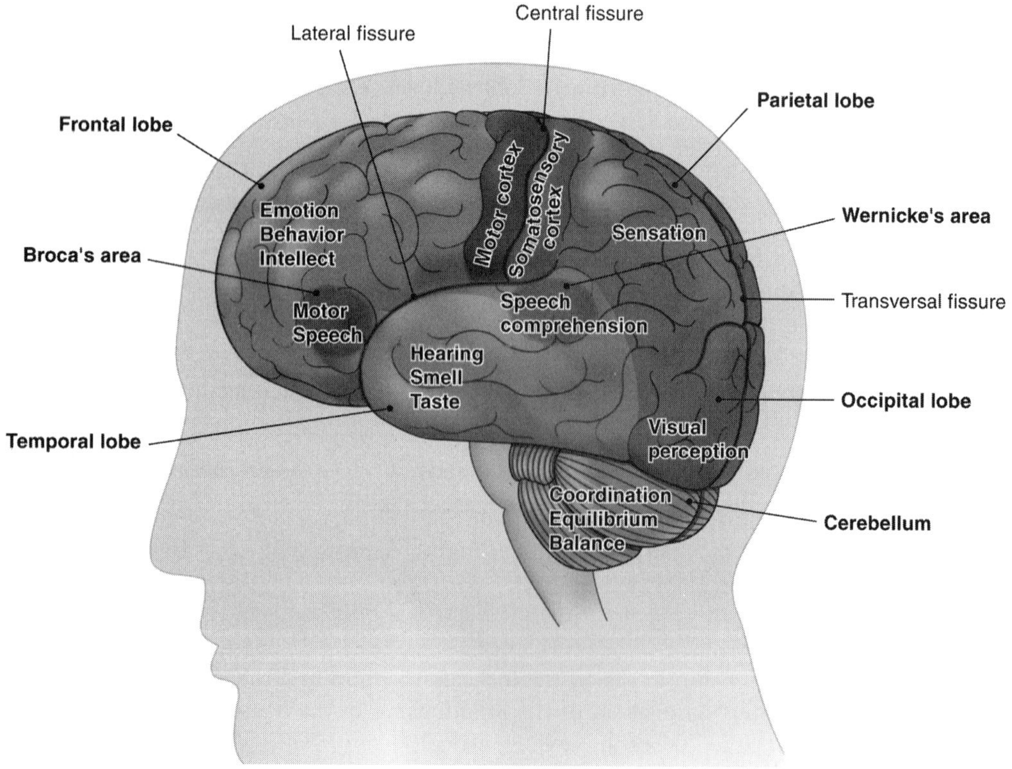

2. 1. b
2. l
3. j
4. c
5. a
6. h
7. f
8. e
9. g
10. k
11. i
12. d

3. Person, place, and time

4. Sternal rub, nail pressure, and Achilles pinch

5. Nipple twist and eyeball pressure

6. Immediate, recent, and remote memory

7. Immediate and recent

8. Psychiatric problem

9. 1. c
2. a
3. b
4. e
5. d
6. j
7. f
8. g
9. h
10. l
11. i
12. k

10. 1. b
2. e
3. d
4. a
5. c

11. Have the patient clench his or her teeth or interlock the hands and push.

12. 0 = Absent; +1 = diminished; +2 = normal; +3 = hyperactive; +4 = hyperactive with clonus.

13. Normal: Toe curling
Abnormal: Fanning of toes and dorsiflexion of great toe

14. Close your eyes.

15. Temperature, because pain and temperature run along the same tract.

16. Yes for deep sensation, no for superficial sensation

17. Have the patient close her or his eyes, then place a vibrating tuning fork on a bony prominence on a finger and a toe.

18. Have the patient close his or her eyes, then move your finger up and down and ask the patient to identify the direction of movement.

19. 1. c
2. e
3. d
4. b
5. a

20. For answers, see "Relationship of the Sensory-Neurologic System to Other Systems," on page 750 of the text, and "Assessment of the Sensory-Neurologic System's Relationship to Other Systems," on page 765 of the text.

21. Increased intracranial pressure

22. A change in level of consciousness

23. Worsening headache, vomiting, sleepy, lethargic, change in Glasgow Coma Scale to 14, change in pupillary reaction (sluggish), change in vital signs, widening pulse pressure, decrease in heart rate, and decrease in motor strength

24. a. Headache and vomiting, change in level of consciousness, change in pupils, and change in vital signs
b. Involved in car accident and sustained concussion, complaints of worsening headache, and guarding head and neck

26. 1. B R (A) I N
2. (C) O R T E X
3. T H A (L) A M U S
4. (S) Y N A P S E
5. A F F (E) R E N T
6. N E U R O N (S)
7. C E R E B E (L) L U M
8. M E D U L L (A)
9. (W) E R N I C K E
10. B R (O) C A' S (A) R E A
11. (G) R A Y (M) A T T E R
12. (C) E R E B R U M
13. M E N I N (G) E S
14. (O) C C I P I T A L L O B E

A C L S E S L A W O A G M C G O
The universal tool used to assess level of consciousness is the GLASGOW COMA SCALE.

Chapter 22: Putting It All Together

1. Cardiovascular examination and TSE

2. HTN, cardiovascular disease, diet (especially cholesterol), and occupational safety

3. Positive: Sought health screening; has supports
Negative: Smoking, alcohol use, high-cholesterol diet, family history of cardiovascular disease, occupational risks, doesn't practice preventive screenings

4. a. Lack of ability to perform TSE
b. Construction worker

Chapter 23: Assessing the Mother-to-Be

1. 1. e
   2. g
   3. l
   4. k
   5. m
   6. h
   7. b
   8. n
   9. a
   10. d
   11. f
   12. c
   13. i
   14. o
   15. j

2. a. Positive
   b. Presumptive
   c. Probable
   d. Presumptive
   e. Probable
   f. Probable
   g. Presumptive
   h. Presumptive
   i. Probable
   j. Probable
   k. Positive
   l. Probable
   m. Presumptive
   n. Presumptive
   o. Presumptive

3. Diabetes, HTN, mitral valve prolapse, hepatitis B, cancer, rubella, and STDs

4. Weight, fundal height, fetal heart tones, and fetal position

5. 7/8/06

6. Breasts, fundus, bleeding, vascular assessment for thrombus, urination, episiotomy or incision, and gastrointestinal problems such as hemorrhoids and bowel movements

7. For answers, see "Normal Changes Associated With Pregnancy," on pages 814-818 of the text.

9. Soft uterus, heavy bleeding, pale color, and vital signs

10. Low BP, increased pulse, pale color, poor capillary refill, skin cool and clammy, soft uterus, and heavy bleeding with clots

11. Shallow respirations, decreased sensation in lower extremities, weakness, and numbness of lower extremities

12. Skin turgor, hydration, mucous membranes, and urinary output

13. The abdomen

14. Supports, prenatal classes, instructions on infant care and breast-feeding, and follow-up care for mother and infant

15. a. Heavy bleeding, low BP, increased pulse, pale color, and cool and clammy skin
    b. Type of anesthesia, hypoventilating, and tender abdominal incision
    c. Cesarean section and surgical incision
    d. Surgery and abdominal incision

Chapter 24 Assessing the Newborn and Infant

1. 1. k
   2. c
   3. a
   4. f
   5. d
   6. e
   7. l
   8. b
   9. j
   10. h
   11. i
   12. g

2. Heart rate, respirations, muscle tone, color, and reflex irritability (cry)

3. Prenatal history; pregnancy, labor, and delivery; anesthesia; type of delivery; medication use during pregnancy (including alcohol, illegal drugs, and over-the-counter [OTC] drugs); medical problems during pregnancy; and prenatal care

4. Head, chest, abdomen, length, and weight

5. 1. d
   2. g
   3. l
   4. b
   5. k
   6. e
   7. f
   8. p
   9. j
   10. m
   11. h
   12. i
   13. c
   14. o
   15. n
   16. a

6. For answers, see "Performing a Newborn Head-to-Toe Physical Assessment," on pages 856-867 of the text.

8. Age—Commonly occurs between 1 and 10 weeks of age
   Gender—More common in boys
   Race—More common in whites than in African Americans or Asians
   Being full-term—More common in full-term infants than in premature infants
   Family history of pyloric stenosis
   Birth order—More common in firstborns

9. How many bowel movements does he have a day? What are their color and consistency?
   How many diaper changes does he need a day for urination?
   How many times a day does he vomit, and how much?
   How many feedings is he able to keep down a day?
10. Vomiting within 1 hour after feeding, projectile vomiting, vomitus described as stale milk, distended upper abdomen, reverse peristaltic waves, and palpable olive-shaped mass in epigastric region
11. Vomiting; weight loss; increase in temperature, pulse, and respirations; sunken fontanels; dry, warm skin and mucous membranes; and lethargic, weak, and inactive
12. Trust versus mistrust
13. Allow mother to stay with child
14. a. Vomiting; increase in vital signs; sunken fontanels; dry, warm skin and mucous membranes; and weight loss
    b. Weight loss and vomiting
15. Secondary to vomiting

Chapter 25 Assessing the Toddler and Preschooler

1. Successful: Gains control over bodily functions, can separate from parents, is able to differentiate self from others, can tolerate delayed gratification.
   Unsuccessful: Feels shame and doubt, has temper tantrums, persistently says "no."
2. Successful: Develops conscience, sees actions as good or bad, motivated by reward or punishment.
   Unsuccessful: Is unable to see actions as good or bad.
3. Toilet training, temper tantrums, and accidents
4. Repeated ED visits, physical findings that are inconsistent with stated cause of injury, inappropriate response by child or parent, inconsistent accounts of injury, other signs of abuse, and evidence of old abuse
5. Allow parent to be with child, use toys or games to demonstrate parts of examination, and do otoscope/ophthalmoscope exam last
6. Need to measure head circumference, plot height and weight on growth charts, assess fontanel, and pull ear lobe down when performing the otoscopic exam
7. For answers, see "Performing a Head-to-Toe Physical Assessment," on pages 893-897 of the text.
9. Low weight and small size for age; 24-hour dietary recall
10. Diet mainly consists of bottles of milk.
11. History of recurrent ear infections, recent upper respiratory infection, his age, bottles at bedtime, and exposure to second-hand smoke
12. Lead paint poisoning; motor vehicle injuries due to improper car seat
13. History of recurrent ear infections, recent upper respiratory infection, fever, tugging at ear, irritable, not sleeping well, decreased appetite, red tympanic membrane, and lymphadenopathy

14. Not active, increased heart rate and respirations, pale conjunctiva, spoon-shaped nails, 24-hour dietary recall shows nutritional deficits, and low hematocrit and hemoglobin
15. Fever, dehydration, and anemia
16. Max's diet, bottles at bedtime, exposure to second-hand smoke, possible lead paint exposure, car safety
17. Autonomy versus shame and doubt
18. Bowel and bladder control
19. 24-hour dietary recall and nutritional deficits
20. a. Temperature elevation: 101.2°F (rectal)
    b. Age, dietary deficits, and anemia
    c. Old house with probable exposure to lead paint, and improper car safety

Chapter 26 Assessing the School-Age Child and Adolescent

1. Successful: Develops independence, learns to work and cooperate with others, builds relationships outside home with peers and teachers, develops a conscience.
   Unsuccessful: Is dependent; fails in school; has difficulty developing relationships; engages in unhealthy, risky behaviors.
2. Successful: Develops a sense of self and self-competency and a set of personal values, plans for future career.
   Unsuccessful: Develops poor self-image, is insecure, engages in unhealthy, risky behaviors.
3. Sports-related injuries, motor vehicle accidents, substance abuse, eating disorders, and sexual activity
4. Substance abuse (drugs, alcohol, and smoking); injuries (use of safety equipment when engaging in sports); automobile/driving safety; nutrition (obesity/eating disorders); and sexuality, including STDs and pregnancy
5. Height and weight are compared on growth charts, and secondary sexual characteristic development is assessed.
6. For answers, see "Performing a Head-to-Toe Physical Assessment," on pages 908-911 of the text.
8. Weakness and fatigue, color pale, mucous membranes pale, increase in pulse, low BP and respirations, positive systolic murmur II/VI, bleeding gums, and bruises
9. Temperature elevation, lymph node enlargement, and fatigue
10. a. Risk for infection related to compromised immune system
    b. Risk for injury related to bone marrow effects
    c. Risk for volume fluid deficit related to bleeding
11. a. Weight loss, loss of appetite, and acute lymphocytic leukemia
    b. Complaints of fatigue
13. Industry versus inferiority
14. Needs to have sense of accomplishments in school and develop relationships outside of home
15. The amount she exercises would lead you to think she has a low lean-to-fat ratio that contributes to amenorrhea.

16. Exercise regimen, and irregular cycles are common for 1 to 2 years after menarche
17. Secondary
18. History of anemia, weight loss
19. Identity versus role diffusion
20. Develop relationships, career choices
21. a. Height in 5 percent and weight in less than 5 percent.
    b. Unaware that exercise pattern has effect on menstrual cycle.

Chapter 27 Assessing the Older Adult

1. Multiple problems with multiple treatments, differing disease presentation in the elderly, and exaggeration of symptoms by patient if he or she is a "health pessimist."
2. Allow more time; ask about hearing problems; speak slowly, clearly, and with a low pitch; redirect, but realize the older patient's need to reminisce.
3. Successful: Satisfaction with life, sense of contributing to society
   Unsuccessful: Depression, alcohol abuse, suicidal
4. Keep environment warm and well lit, but use nonglaring light; keep background noise down; use higher than standard seating for patient; and minimize position changes.
5. For answers, see "Performing a Head-to-Toe Physical Assessment," on pages 949-956 of the text.
6. 1. b
   2. c
   3. d
   4. a
8. Integrity versus despair
9. The pain and decreased ability to be active could lead to depression.
10. Rheumatoid arthritis is systemic, with associated symptoms of fatigue and fever.
11. Age, occupation, and weight
12. Pain with movement, limited ROM, gait problems, crepitus, decreased strength, and swelling of knees
13. a. Pain increases with activity.
    b. Knee pain, decreased ROM, needs cane to walk, and decreased strength.
    c. Reports awakening at night with knee pain.

Apea
contact ASK
800-899 4502